*Quick*FACTS™

Colorectal
CANCER

What You Need to Know—NOW

SECOND EDITION

*Quick*FACTS™

From the Experts at the American Cancer Society

Colorectal
CANCER

What You Need to Know—NOW

SECOND EDITION

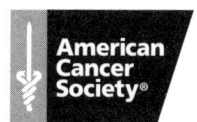

Published by the American Cancer Society/Health Promotions
250 Williams Street NW, Atlanta, Georgia 30303 USA

Copyright ©2008 American Cancer Society

Printed in the United States of America
Cover designed by Jill Dible, Atlanta, GA

5 4 3 2 1   08 09 10 11 12

Library of Congress Cataloging-in-Publication Data

Quick facts colorectal cancer : what you need to know—now / from the experts at the American Cancer Society. — 2nd ed.
    p. cm. — (Quick facts)
    Rev. ed. of: Quick facts colon cancer. 2007.
    Includes bibliographical references and index.
    ISBN-13: 978-1-60443-007-3 (pbk. : alk. paper)
    ISBN-10: 1-60443-007-9 (pbk. : alk. paper)
    1. Colon (Anatomy)—Cancer—Popular works.
2. Rectum—Cancer—Popular works. I. American Cancer Society. II. Quick facts colon cancer. III. Title: Colorectal cancer.
    RC280.C6Q53 2008
    616.99'4347—dc22

                                                    2008019967

A Note to the Reader

This information represents the views of the doctors and nurses serving on the American Cancer Society's Cancer Information Database Editorial Board. These views are based on their interpretation of studies published in medical journals, as well as their own professional experience.

The treatment information in this book is not official policy of the Society and is not intended as medical advice to replace the expertise and judgment of your cancer care team. It is intended to help you and your family make informed decisions, together with your doctor.

Your doctor may have reasons for suggesting a treatment plan different from these general treatment options. Don't hesitate to ask your doctor about your treatment options.

For more information, contact your American Cancer Society at **800-ACS-2345** or **http://www.cancer.org**.

Bulk purchases of this book are available at a discount. For information, contact the American Cancer Society at **trade.sales@cancer.org**.

TABLE OF CONTENTS

Your Colorectal Cancer

What Is Cancer?.................................1

What Is Colorectal Cancer? 3

The Normal Digestive System 3

Abnormal Growths in the Colon or Rectum 5

Start and Spread of Colorectal Cancer.............6

Types of Cancer in the Colon and Rectum 7

What Are the Key Statistics About
Colorectal Cancer? 8

Risk Factors and Causes

What Are the Risk Factors for
Colorectal Cancer? 11

Risk Factors You Cannot Change 12

Lifestyle-Related Factors 16

Factors with Uncertain or Unproven Effects on
Colorectal Cancer 18

Do We Know What Causes
Colorectal Cancer? 19

Inherited Gene Mutations 20

Acquired Gene Mutations 21

Prevention and Detection

Can Colorectal Cancer Be Prevented?...........23

Screening....................................23

Genetic Testing and Screening for Those
with a Strong Family History....................24

Diet, Exercise, and Body Weight 27

Vitamins, Calcium, and Magnesium 29

Nonsteroidal Anti-inflammatory Drugs 30

Hormone Replacement Therapy 31

Can Colorectal Polyps and Cancer Be Found Early? 31

Types of Colorectal Cancer Screening Tests 31

Screening Tests That Can Find Both Colorectal Polyps and Cancer 32

Screening Tests That Mainly Find Colorectal Cancer 42

Pros and Cons of Various Screening Tests 49

American Cancer Society Recommendations for Colorectal Cancer Early Detection 51

People at Average Risk 51

People at Increased or High Risk 52

American Cancer Society Guidelines on Screening and Surveillance for the Early Detection of Colorectal Adenomas and Cancer in People at Increased Risk or High Risk 54

Insurance Coverage for Colorectal Cancer Screening 58

Diagnosis and Staging

How Is Colorectal Cancer Diagnosed? 59

Signs and Symptoms of Colorectal Cancer 59

Medical History and Physical Examination 60

Blood Tests 60

Tests to Detect Colorectal Polyps or Cancer 62

Biopsy 62

Imaging Tests 62

How Is Colorectal Cancer Staged? 68

AJCC (TNM) Staging System 69

Stage Grouping 72

Comparison of AJCC, Dukes, and
Astler-Coller Stages 74

Survival Rates for Colorectal Cancer. 75
Survival Rates for Colon Cancer, by Stage. 75
Relative Survival Rates for Rectal Cancer, by Stage . . .76

Grade of Colorectal Cancer. 77

Treatments

Your Medical Team 79
Dietitian. 79
Gastroenterologist 79
Genetic Counselor. 81
Medical Oncologist 81
Nurses 81
Pain Specialist 82
Pathologist. 83
Personal or Primary Care Physician. 83
Physician Assistant. 83
Psychologist or Psychiatrist 84
Radiation Oncologist 84
Radiologist. 84
Social Worker 85
Surgeon 85
Urologist 86

How Is Colorectal Cancer Treated? 86
Making Treatment Decisions .87

Surgery. 87
Colon Surgery 88
Rectal Surgery 90
Side Effects of Colorectal Surgery 93
Surgical Treatment of Colorectal
Cancer Metastases 96

Radiation Therapy **98**

   Types of Radiation Therapy 99

   Side Effects of Radiation Therapy 100

Chemotherapy **101**

   Drugs Used to Treat Colorectal Cancer 103

   Side Effects of Chemotherapy 105

Targeted Therapies **107**

Treatment by Stage of Colon Cancer **109**

   Treatment for Stage 0 Colon Cancer 109

   Treatment for Stage I Colon Cancer. 110

   Treatment for Stage II Colon Cancer 110

   Treatment for Stage III Colon Cancer 111

   Treatment for Stage IV Colon Cancer 111

   Treatment for Recurrent Colon Cancer 113

Treatment by Stage of Rectal Cancer **114**

   Treatment for Stage 0 Rectal Cancer 114

   Treatment for Stage I Rectal Cancer. 115

   Treatment for Stage II Rectal Cancer 115

   Treatment for Stage III Rectal Cancer 116

   Treatment for Stage IV Rectal Cancer 117

   Treatment for Recurrent Rectal Cancer 119

Clinical Trials **121**

   What Are Clinical Trials? 121

   Phases of Clinical Trials 122

   Taking Part in a Clinical Trial 124

   How Can I Find Out More About Clinical
Trials That Might Be Right for Me? 126

Complementary and Alternative Therapies **127**

   Considering Your Options. 129

More Treatment Information **131**

Questions to Ask

What Should You Ask Your Doctor About
Colorectal Cancer? 133

After Treatment

What Happens After Treatment for
Colorectal Cancer? 135
Follow-up Care 135
For Patients with a Colostomy. 137
Seeing a New Doctor. 137

Lifestyle Changes to Consider During and
After Treatment 138
Make Healthier Choices. 139
Diet and Nutrition. 139
Rest, Fatigue, Work, and Exercise 140

Can You Reduce Your Risk for
Cancer Recurrence?. 142
Physical Activity. 143
Diet 143

How About Your Emotional Health? 143

What Happens If Treatment Is No
Longer Working? 145

Latest Research

What's New in Colorectal Cancer Research
and Treatment? 149
Genetics. 149
Chemoprevention 149
Earlier Detection 151
Treatment. 152

Resources

Additional Resources **155**

    More Information from Your American
    Cancer Society. 155

    National Organizations and Web Sites. 156

    References 157

Glossary   **161**

Index   **191**

Your Colorectal Cancer

What Is Cancer?

Cancer* develops when **cells** in a part of the body begin to grow out of control. Although there are many kinds of cancer, they all start because of out-of-control growth of abnormal cells.

Normal body cells grow, divide, and die in an orderly fashion. During the early years of a person's life, normal cells divide rapidly. After the person becomes an adult, cells in most parts of the body divide only to replace worn-out or dying cells and to repair injuries.

Because **cancer cells** continue to grow and divide, they are different from normal cells. Instead of dying in the expected time frame, cancer cells outlive normal cells and continue to form new abnormal cells.

Cancer cells develop because of damage to **DNA.** DNA is in every cell and directs all the cell's activities. Most of the time when DNA becomes damaged, the body is able to repair it. In cancer

*Terms in **bold type** are further explained in the Glossary, beginning on page 161.

cells, the damaged DNA is not repaired. People can inherit damaged DNA, which accounts for inherited cancer. Many times though, a person's DNA becomes damaged by exposure to something in the environment, like smoke.

Cancer usually forms as a **tumor.** Some types of cancer, like leukemia, do not form tumors. Instead, these cancer cells involve the blood and blood-forming organs and circulate through other tissues where they grow.

Often, cancer cells travel to other parts of the body, where they begin to grow and replace normal **tissue.** This process is called **metastasis.** Regardless of where a cancer may spread, however, it is always named for the place it began. For instance, breast cancer that spreads to the **liver** is still called breast cancer, not liver cancer.

Not all tumors are cancerous. **Benign** (noncancerous) tumors do not spread (**metastasize**) to other parts of the body and, with very rare exceptions, are not life-threatening.

Different types of cancer can behave very differently. For example, lung cancer and breast cancer are very different diseases. They grow at different rates and respond to different treatments. That is why people with cancer need treatment that is aimed at their particular kind of cancer.

Cancer is the second leading cause of death in the United States. Cancer will develop in nearly half of all men and a little over one-third of all women in the United States during their lifetimes. Today, millions of people are living with cancer or have had cancer. The risk for developing most types of cancer can be reduced by changes in a person's lifestyle; for example, by quitting smoking and eating a better diet. The sooner a cancer is found and treatment begun, the better the chances are for living many years.

What Is Colorectal Cancer?

Colorectal cancer refers to cancer that develops in the **colon** or the **rectum.** Colorectal cancer is sometimes referred to separately as colon cancer or rectal cancer, depending on where it starts. Colon cancer and rectal cancer have many features in common. They are discussed together in this book except for the chapter on treatment, in which they are discussed separately.

The Normal Digestive System

The colon and rectum are parts of the **digestive system,** which is also called the **gastrointestinal (GI) tract** (see picture on page 5). In order to understand colorectal cancer, it helps to have some basic knowledge about the normal structure and function of the digestive system.

After food is chewed and swallowed, it travels through the **esophagus** to the **stomach.** There it is partly broken down and then sent to the **small intestine** (also known as the small **bowel**). The word "small" refers to the diameter of the small intestine, which is narrower than that of the large bowel (colon and rectum). Actually, the small intestine is the longest segment of the digestive system—about 20 feet. The small intestine continues breaking down the food and absorbs most of the nutrients.

The small intestine joins the colon in the right lower **abdomen**. The colon (also called the large bowel or **large intestine**) is a muscular tube about 5 feet long. The colon absorbs water and salt from food matter and serves as a storage place for waste matter.

The colon has 4 sections:

- The first section is called the **ascending colon.** It starts with a small pouch (the cecum) where the small bowel attaches to the colon and extends upward on the right side of the abdomen. The **cecum** is also where the **appendix** attaches to the colon.
- The second section is called the **transverse colon;** it goes across the body from the right to the left side in the upper abdomen.
- The third section, the **descending colon,** continues downward on the left side.
- The fourth and last section is known as the **sigmoid colon** because of its "S" or "sigmoid" shape.

The waste matter that is left after going through the colon is known as **feces** or **stool.** It goes into the **rectum,** the final 6 inches of the digestive system. From there it passes out of the body through the **anus.**

The wall of the colon and rectum is made up of several layers of tissue. Colorectal cancer starts in the innermost layer and can grow through some or

The Digestive System

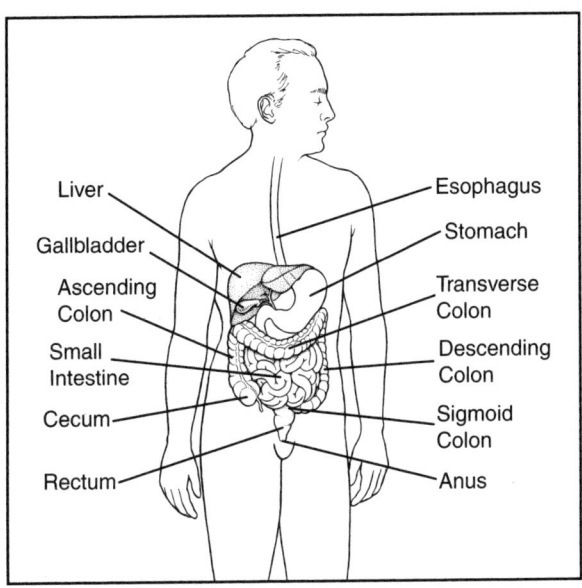

Liver

Gallbladder

Ascending Colon

Small Intestine

Cecum

Rectum

Esophagus

Stomach

Transverse Colon

Descending Colon

Sigmoid Colon

Anus

all of the other layers. Knowing a little about these layers is important, because the **stage** (extent of spread) of a colorectal cancer depends to a great degree on how deeply it invades into these layers. For more information, see the section on staging, beginning on page 68.

Abnormal Growths in the Colon or Rectum

In most people, colorectal cancer develops slowly over a period of several years. Before a cancer develops, a growth or tumor usually develops on the inner lining of the colon or rectum. A tumor is abnormal tissue and can be benign (noncancerous) or **malignant** (cancerous). A **polyp** is a benign, noncancerous tumor. Some polyps can change into cancer but not all do. The likelihood that a polyp will change into cancer depends on the kind of polyp:

- **Adenomatous polyps (adenomas)** are polyps that have the potential to change into cancer. Because of this, adenomas represent a **precancerous** condition.
- **Hyperplastic polyps** and **inflammatory polyps,** in general, are not precancerous. Some doctors think that some hyperplastic polyps can become precancerous or might be a sign the person is at greater risk of developing adenomas and cancer, particularly when these polyps grow in the ascending colon.

Another kind of precancerous condition is called **dysplasia.** When dysplasia develops in the lining of the colon or rectum, the cells look abnormal (but not like true cancer cells) when viewed under a microscope. These cells have the potential to change into cancer over time. Dysplasia is usually seen in people who have had diseases such as **ulcerative colitis** or **Crohn's disease** for many years. Both ulcerative colitis and Crohn's disease cause chronic inflammation of the colon.

Start and Spread of Colorectal Cancer

If cancer forms within a polyp, it can eventually begin to grow into the wall of the colon or rectum. When cancer cells are in the wall, they can then grow into blood vessels or lymphatic vessels.

Lymphatic vessels are thin, tiny channels that carry away waste and fluid. They first drain into nearby **lymph nodes,** which are bean-shaped structures that help fight against infections. Once cancer cells spread into blood or lymphatic vessels, they can travel to distant parts of the body, such as the liver. This process of spread is called metastasis.

Types of Cancer in the Colon and Rectum

Adenocarcinoma

More than 95% of colorectal cancer is of a type of cancer known as **adenocarcinoma.** Adenocarcinoma starts in cells that form the glands that make **mucus** to lubricate the inside of the colon and rectum. When doctors talk about colorectal cancer, adenocarcinoma is almost always the type to which they are referring. This book focuses on colorectal adenocarcinoma.

Other, less common types of tumors may also develop in the colon and rectum:

Carcinoid tumors

Carcinoid tumors develop from specialized hormone-producing cells of the intestine. For more information on these tumors, call the American Cancer Society at **800-ACS-2345** and ask for the document *Gastrointestinal Carcinoid Tumors,* or look online at **www.cancer.org.**

Gastrointestinal stromal tumors (GISTs)

Gastrointestinal stromal tumors (GISTs) develop from specialized cells in the wall of the colon called the "interstitial cells of Cajal." Some are benign (noncancerous); others are malignant (cancerous). Although these tumors can be found anywhere in the digestive tract, they are unusual in the colon. For more information on these tumors, call the American Cancer Society at **800-ACS-2345** and ask for the document *Gastrointestinal Stromal Tumors,* or look online at **www.cancer.org.**

Lymphoma

Lymphoma is a cancer of the immune system cells. It typically develops in lymph nodes, but it may also start in the colon and rectum or other organs. For more information on lymphoma, call the American Cancer Society at **800-ACS-2345** and ask for the document *Non-Hodgkin Lymphoma,* or look online at **www.cancer.org.**

What Are the Key Statistics About Colorectal Cancer?

Excluding skin cancer, colorectal cancer is the third most common cancer diagnosed in both men and women in the United States. The American Cancer Society estimates that about 108,070 new cases of colon cancer (53,760 in men and 54,310 in women) and 40,740 new cases of rectal cancer (23,490 in men and 17,250 in women) will be diagnosed in 2008.

The lifetime risk for developing colorectal cancer is about 1 in 19 (5.4%). This risk is slightly higher in men than in women. A number of other factors may also affect a person's risk. These factors are discussed in the next chapter.

Colorectal cancer is the third leading cause of cancer-related deaths in the United States when men and women are considered separately, and the second leading cause when both sexes are combined. It is expected to cause about 49,960 deaths (24,260 men and 25,700 women) during 2008.

The death rate (the number of deaths per 100,000 people per year) from colorectal cancer has been dropping for more than 20 years. There are a number of likely reasons for this decline. One is that polyps are being found by screening and removed before they can develop into cancer. Screening is also allowing more colorectal cancers to be found earlier when the disease is easier to cure. In addition, treatment for colorectal cancer has improved over the last several years. As a result, there are now more than 1 million survivors of colorectal cancer in the United States.

Risk Factors and Causes

What Are the Risk Factors for Colorectal Cancer?

A **risk factor** is anything that affects your chance of getting a disease such as cancer. Different types of cancer have different risk factors. For example, exposing skin to strong sunlight is a risk factor for skin cancer, and smoking is a risk factor for cancer of the lungs, larynx, mouth, throat, esophagus, kidneys, bladder, colon, and several other organs.

Risk factors do not tell us everything. Having a risk factor, or even several risk factors, does not mean that you will get the disease. Some people who get the disease may not have any known risk factors. Even if a person with colorectal cancer has a risk factor, it is often very hard to know how much that risk factor may have contributed to the cancer.

Researchers have found several risk factors that may increase the chance that colorectal polyps or colorectal cancer will develop.

Risk Factors You Cannot Change

Age

Whereas younger adults may have a diagnosis of colorectal cancer, the chances of developing colorectal cancer increase markedly after age 50. More than 90% of colorectal cancer diagnoses are in people older than 50.

Personal history of colorectal polyps or colorectal cancer

If you have a history of adenomatous polyps (adenomas), you are at increased risk for colorectal cancer. This is especially true if the polyps are large or if there are many of them.

If you have had colorectal cancer, even though it has been completely removed, this increases the likelihood that new cancer will develop in other areas of the colon and rectum. The chances of this happening are greater if you had your first colorectal cancer diagnosis when you were younger than age 60.

Personal history of inflammatory bowel disease

Inflammatory bowel disease (IBD), which includes ulcerative colitis and Crohn's disease, is a condition in which the colon is inflamed over a long period. If you have IBD, your risk of colorectal cancer developing is increased, and you need to be screened for colorectal cancer on a more frequent basis (see "Can Colorectal Polyps and Cancer Be Found Early?" on page 31). Often, the first **sign** that cancer may be developing is dysplasia, which refers to abnormal cells that have the potential to progress to cancer.

Inflammatory bowel disease is different from **irritable bowel syndrome (IBS),** which does not carry an increased risk for colorectal cancer.

Family history of colorectal cancer

Most instances of colorectal cancer occur in people without a family history of colorectal cancer. Still, up to 20% of people who have colorectal cancer have other family members who have also been affected by this disease.

If a person has a **first-degree relative** (parent, sibling, or child) with a history of colorectal cancer or adenomatous polyps, that person is at increased risk for colorectal cancer. The risk is about doubled in those with just one affected first-degree relative. The risk is higher in people with a stronger family history, such as in these circumstances:

- a history of colorectal cancer or adenomatous polyps in any first-degree relative who was younger than age 60 at the time of diagnosis
- a history of colorectal cancer or adenomatous polyps in 2 or more first-degree relatives at any age

Why family history increases risk is not clear in all cases. Cancer can "run in the family" because of inherited genes, shared environmental factors, or some combination of these factors.

People diagnosed with adenomatous polyps or colorectal cancer should inform other family members. Those with a family history of colorectal cancer need to talk with their doctor about the possible need to begin screening before age 50.

Inherited syndromes

About 5% of people who receive a diagnosis of colorectal cancer have an inherited genetic susceptibility to the disease. The 2 most common inherited syndromes linked with colorectal cancer are **familial adenomatous polyposis** (FAP) and **hereditary nonpolyposis colon cancer** (HNPCC).

Familial adenomatous polyposis (FAP) is caused by changes, or mutations, in a **gene** called the **APC gene.** A person inherits the APC gene from his or her parents. About 1% of all colorectal cancer is due to FAP. Typically, hundreds or thousands of polyps develop in the colon and rectum of people with this disease, usually in their teens or early adulthood. Cancer usually develops in one or more of these polyps as early as age 20. Cancer will develop in almost all people with this disorder by the age of 40 unless preventive surgery (removal of the colon) is done. FAP is sometimes associated with **Gardner syndrome,** a condition that involves benign tumors of the skin, soft connective tissue, and bones.

Another clearly defined genetic syndrome is hereditary nonpolyposis colon cancer (HNPCC), also known as **Lynch syndrome.** It accounts for about 3% to 4% of all colorectal cancer. HNPCC can be caused by inherited changes in a number of different genes that normally help repair DNA damage. This syndrome also develops when people are relatively young. People with HNPCC have polyps, but they have only a few, not hundreds as with FAP. The lifetime risk for colorectal cancer in people with this condition may be as high as 70% to 80%.

Women with HNPCC also have a very high risk of developing cancer of the endometrium (the lining of the uterus). Other types of cancer linked with HNPCC include cancer of the ovary, stomach, small bowel, pancreas, kidney, ureters (the tubes that carry urine from the kidneys to the bladder), and bile duct.

People with the rare inherited condition **Peutz-Jeghers syndrome** tend to have large polyps in their digestive tracts and dark spots around the mouth and on the hands and feet. They are at greatly increased risk for colorectal cancer, as well as several other types of cancer, which usually appear at an age well below the average.

Inherited gene mutations are discussed further on pages 20–21. Identifying families with these inherited syndromes is important because it allows doctors to recommend specific steps, such as **screening** and other preventive measures, when patients are younger. Because several types of cancer can be linked with these syndromes, people should check their family medical histories for polyps or any type of cancer. Those who have polyps or cancer should inform other family members. People with a family history of colorectal polyps or cancer should consider **genetic counseling** to review their family medical tree and determine whether **genetic testing** may be right for them.

If needed, this can help them to decide about getting screened and treated at an early age. More information on genetic counseling and testing can be found on pages 24–27.

Racial and ethnic background

African Americans have the highest colorectal cancer incidence and mortality rates of all racial groups in the United States. The reason for this disparity is not yet understood.

Jews of Eastern European descent (Ashkenazi Jews) have one of the highest colorectal cancer risks of any ethnic group in the world. Several gene mutations leading to an increased risk of colorectal cancer have been found in this group. The most common of these DNA changes, called the I1307K APC mutation, is present in about 6% of American Jews.

Lifestyle-Related Factors

Several lifestyle-related factors have been linked to colorectal cancer. In fact, the links between diet, weight, and exercise and colorectal cancer risk are some of the strongest for any type of cancer.

Certain types of diets

A diet that is high in red meats (beef, lamb, or liver) and processed meats (hot dogs, bologna, and luncheon meat) can increase colorectal cancer risk. Methods of cooking meats at very high temperatures (frying, broiling, or grilling) create chemicals that might increase cancer risk, although it is not clear how much this might contribute to an increase in colorectal cancer risk. Diets high in vegetables and fruits have been linked with a decreased risk of colorectal cancer. Whether other dietary components (such as **fiber** or certain types of fats) affect colorectal cancer risk is not clear.

Physical inactivity

If you are not physically active, you have a greater chance of developing colorectal cancer. Increasing activity may help reduce your risk.

Obesity

The risk for colorectal cancer to develop and cause death is increased in very overweight people. Whereas obesity raises the risk of colon cancer in both men and women, the link seems to be stronger in men.

Smoking

Colorectal cancer is more likely to develop and cause death in long-term smokers than in nonsmokers. Whereas smoking is a well-known cause of lung cancer, some of the cancer-causing substances released during smoking are swallowed and can cause digestive system cancers, such as colorectal cancer.

Heavy alcohol use

Colorectal cancer has been linked to the heavy use of alcohol. At least some of this may be due to the fact that heavy alcohol users tend to have low levels of **folic acid** in the body. Still, alcohol use should be limited to no more than 2 drinks a day for men and 1 drink a day for women.

Type 2 Diabetes

People with type 2 (usually non–insulin-dependent) diabetes are at increased risk for colorectal cancer. Type 2 diabetes and colorectal cancer share some of the same risk factors (such as excess weight). But even after taking these into account, people with type 2 diabetes still have an increased risk. They also tend to have a less favorable **prognosis** (outlook) after diagnosis.

Factors with Uncertain or Unproven Effects on Colorectal Cancer

Night-shift work

Results of one study suggest that working a night shift at least 3 nights a month for at least 15 years may increase the risk for colorectal cancer in women. The study authors suggested this might be due to changes in levels of **melatonin** (a hormone that responds to changes in light) in the body. More research is needed to confirm or refute this finding.

Previous treatment for certain types of cancer

Some studies have found that men who survive testicular cancer seem to have a higher rate of colorectal cancer and some other types of cancer. This might be due to the treatments they have received.

Some early studies suggested that men who received radiation therapy to treat prostate cancer might have a higher risk of rectal cancer, because the rectum receives some radiation during treatment. However, other studies have not found such a link.

The American Cancer Society and several other medical organizations recommend earlier screening for people with increased risk for colorectal cancer. These recommendations differ from those for people at average risk. For more information, speak with your doctor and refer to the table on page 54.

Do We Know What Causes Colorectal Cancer?

Although we do not know the exact cause of most colorectal cancer, there is a great deal of research in this area. Researchers are beginning to understand how certain changes in DNA can cause normal cells to become cancerous. DNA is the chemical in each of our cells that makes up our genes—the instructions for how our cells function. We usually resemble our parents because they are the source of our DNA. However, DNA affects more than just how we look. Some genes contain instructions for controlling when our cells grow, divide, and die. Certain genes that speed up cell division are called **oncogenes.** Others that slow down cell division, or cause cells to die at the right time, are called **tumor suppressor genes.** Cancer can be caused by DNA mutations that "turn on" oncogenes or "turn off" tumor suppressor genes. Changes in several different genes seem to be needed to cause colorectal cancer.

DNA mutations may be passed on from generation to generation. When this happens, we say the mutations are inherited. Other mutations happen during an individual's lifetime and are not passed on. These DNA changes are called acquired mutations. These are the most common type of mutations. Some of the same genes are involved in both hereditary and acquired mutations.

Inherited Gene Mutations

A small percentage of colorectal cancer cases are known to be caused by inherited gene mutations. Many of these DNA changes and their effects on how cell growth is controlled are now known.

Inherited changes in a gene called APC, for example, are responsible for familial adenomatous polyposis (FAP) and Gardner syndrome. The APC gene is a tumor suppressor gene—it normally helps keep cell growth in check. In people who have inherited changes in the APC gene, this "brake" on cell growth is turned off, resulting in the formation of hundreds of polyps in the colon. Over time, cancer will nearly always develop in one or more of these polyps because new gene mutations occur in the cells of the polyps.

Hereditary nonpolyposis colon cancer (HNPCC), also known as Lynch syndrome, is caused by changes in genes that normally help a cell repair faulty DNA. Cells must make a new copy of their DNA each time they divide. Sometimes errors are made when copying the DNA code. Fortunately, cells have DNA repair enzymes that act like proofreaders. Mutations in DNA repair enzyme genes such as MLH1, MSH2, MSH6, or PMS2 allow DNA errors to go uncorrected. These errors will sometimes affect growth-regulating genes, which may lead to the development of cancer.

The rare Peutz-Jeghers syndrome is caused by inherited changes in the STK11 gene. The STK11 gene seems to be a tumor suppressor gene, although its exact function is not clear.

Genetic tests are available that can detect gene mutations associated with these inherited syndromes. As mentioned earlier, people with a family history of colorectal polyps or cancer or other symptoms linked to these syndromes may want to ask their doctor about genetic counseling and genetic testing. The American Cancer Society recommends discussing genetic testing with a qualified genetic counselor before genetic testing is done.

Acquired Gene Mutations

In most cases of colorectal cancer, the DNA mutations that lead to cancer are acquired during a person's life rather than having been inherited. While certain risk factors likely play a role in causing these acquired mutations, so far the cause of most of these mutations remains unknown.

There does not seem to be a single pathway to colorectal cancer that is the same in all cases. In many cases, the first mutation occurs in the APC gene. This leads to an increased growth of colorectal cells because of the loss of this "brake" on cell growth. Further mutations may then occur in genes such as K-Ras, p53, and SMAD4. These changes can lead the cells to grow and spread uncontrollably. Other, as of yet unknown genes are likely involved as well.

Prevention and Detection

Can Colorectal Cancer Be Prevented?

Even though we do not know the exact cause of most colorectal cancer, it is often possible to prevent it.

Screening

Regular colorectal cancer screening or testing is one of the most powerful weapons in preventing colorectal cancer. From the time the first abnormal cells start to grow, it usually takes about 10 to 15 years for them to develop into colorectal cancer. In many cases, regular colorectal cancer screening can prevent colorectal cancer altogether. This is because some polyps can be found and removed before they have the chance to turn into cancer. Screening can also result in finding colorectal cancer early, when it is highly curable.

People who have no identified risk factors (other than age) should begin regular screening at age 50. Those who have a family history or other risk factors for colorectal polyps or cancer, such as inflammatory bowel disease, should talk with their doctor about starting screening at a younger age and/or getting screened more often than people of average risk. See the American Cancer Society screening guidelines on page 51 for more information.

Genetic Testing and Screening for Those with a Strong Family History

People with a strong family history of colorectal polyps or cancer should consider genetic counseling to review their family medical tree and determine whether genetic testing may be right for them. If needed, this can help them to decide whether to get screened and treated at an early age.

Before getting genetic testing, it is important to know ahead of time what the results may or may not tell you about your risk. Genetic testing is not perfect and, in some cases, the tests may not be able to provide solid answers. This is why meeting with a genetic counselor before testing is crucial in deciding whether testing should be done.

Genetic tests can help determine whether members of certain families have inherited a high risk for developing colorectal cancer because of syndromes such as familial adenomatous polyposis (FAP) or hereditary nonpolyposis colon cancer (HNPCC). Without genetic testing, all members of a family known to have an inherited form of colorectal cancer should be screened early and frequently. If genetic testing is done for a known mutation within a family, those members who have not inherited the mutated gene may be able to be screened with the same frequency as people at average risk.

To help you decide whether testing might be appropriate for you, a genetic counselor will try to get a detailed view of your family history. For example, doctors have found that many families with HNPCC tend to have certain characteristics:

- at least 3 relatives have colorectal cancer
- of those, one is a first-degree relative (parent, sibling, or child) of one or both of the other 2
- at least 2 successive generations are involved
- at least one relative had cancer before the age of 50

The characteristics listed above are called the **Amsterdam criteria.** If these are true for your family, then you might want to seek genetic counseling. Even if your family history meets the Amsterdam criteria, it does not always mean you have HNPCC. Only about half of families who meet the Amsterdam criteria have HNPCC. The other half do not, and although their colorectal cancer rate is about twice as high as normal, it is not as high as that of people with HNPCC. On the other hand, many families with HNPCC do not meet the Amsterdam criteria.

A second set of criteria, called the **Bethesda Guidelines** (formerly the Bethesda Criteria), are used to determine whether a person with colorectal cancer should have his or her cancer tested for genetic changes that are seen with HNPCC. If a person has colorectal cancer and meets at least one of the criteria below, he or she should consider genetic testing:

- The person is younger than 50 years.
- The person has or had a second colorectal cancer or another cancer of one of the types associated with HNPCC (endometrial, stomach, pancreas, small intestine, ovary, kidney or ureters, bile duct).
- The person is younger than 60 years and the cancer has certain characteristics seen with HNPCC when viewed under the microscope or with other laboratory tests.
- The person has a first-degree relative younger than 50 who had colorectal cancer or another cancer often seen in HNPCC carriers (endometrial, stomach, pancreas, small intestine, ovary, kidney, ureters, or bile duct).
- The person has 2 or more first- or **second-degree relatives** who had colorectal cancer or an HNPCC-related cancer at any age.

If a person with colorectal cancer meets any of the Bethesda guidelines, genetic testing is advised to look for an inherited HNPCC–associated gene mutation. Still, most people who meet the Bethesda guidelines do not have HNPCC.

Not all families with HNPCC meet the criteria above. Doctors should be suspicious of HNPCC in families with colorectal cancer and other types of cancer associated with this syndrome, including endometrial cancer, ovarian cancer, small bowel cancer, pancreatic cancer, or cancer of the lining of the kidney or the ureters.

For people with HNPCC, the lifetime risk for colorectal cancer to develop may be as high as 80%. In families known to carry an HNPCC gene mutation, doctors recommend that family members who have tested positive for the mutation and those who have not been tested start colonoscopy screening during their early 20s to remove any polyps and find any cancer at the earliest possible stage (see the section, "Can colorectal polyps or cancer be found early?" on page 31). People known to carry one of the gene mutations may also be offered the option of having most of the colon removed.

Genetic counseling and testing are also available for those at risk of FAP. For a person with FAP, the lifetime risk for colorectal cancer to develop is near 100% and, in most cases, it develops before the age of 40. People who test positive for the gene change linked to FAP should start colonoscopy screening during their teens (see the section, "Can colorectal polyps or cancer be found early?" on page 31). Most doctors recommend that patients who test positive for FAP have their colon removed when they are in their 20s to prevent cancer from developing.

Diet, Exercise, and Body Weight

People can lower their risk for colorectal cancer by managing the risk factors that they can control, such as diet and physical activity.

Diets high in vegetables and fruits have been linked with a lower risk of colorectal cancer, and diets high in processed and/or red meats have been linked with a higher risk. The American Cancer Society recommends the following:

- Eat a healthy diet, with an emphasis on plant sources.
- Choose foods and beverages in amounts that help achieve and maintain a healthy weight.
- Eat 5 or more servings of a variety of vegetables and fruits each day.
- Choose whole grains rather than processed (refined) grains.
- Limit consumption of processed and red meats.

Physical activity is another area that people can control. The American Cancer Society recommends at least 30 minutes, preferably 45 to 60 minutes, of physical activity on 5 or more days of the week. Taking part in moderate or vigorous activity for 45 minutes on 5 or more days of the week may lower your risk for colorectal cancer even more.

Obesity raises the risk of colorectal cancer in both men and women, but the link seems to be stronger in men. The American Cancer Society recommends that people try to maintain a healthy weight throughout life by balancing what they eat with physical activity. If you are overweight, you can ask your doctor about a weight loss plan that will work for you.

For more information about diet and physical activity, the American Cancer Society's *Guidelines for Nutrition and Physical Activity for Cancer Prevention* are available on the Web at **www.cancer.org** or by calling **800-ACS-2345.**

Vitamins, Calcium, and Magnesium

Some studies suggest that taking a daily multivitamin containing folic acid, or folate, may lower colorectal cancer risk, but not all studies have found this. More research is needed in this area.

Some studies have suggested that vitamin D, which you can get from sun exposure, in food, or in a vitamin pill, can lower colorectal cancer risk. Because of concerns that excessive sun exposure can cause skin cancer, most experts do not recommend this as a way to lower colorectal cancer risk at this time.

Other studies suggest that increasing calcium intake may lower colorectal cancer risk. Calcium is important for a number of health reasons aside from possible effects on cancer risk. However, because of the possible increased risk of prostate cancer with high calcium intake, it may be wise for men to limit their daily calcium intake to less than 1500 mg per day until further studies are done.

Calcium and vitamin D may work together to reduce colorectal cancer risk, as vitamin D aids in the body's absorption of calcium. Still, not all studies have found that these nutrients reduce risk.

A few studies have looked at a possible link between a diet high in magnesium and reduced colorectal cancer risk. Some, but not all, of these studies have found a link, especially among women.

More research is needed to determine whether this link exists.

Nonsteroidal Anti-inflammatory Drugs

Many studies have found that people who regularly use aspirin and other **nonsteroidal anti-inflammatory drugs (NSAIDs),** such as ibuprofen (Motrin, Advil) and naproxen (Aleve), have a lower risk for colorectal cancer and adenomatous polyps. Most of these studies looked at people who took these medicines for arthritis or prevention of heart attacks. Other, stronger studies have provided evidence that aspirin can prevent the growth of polyps in people who were previously treated for early stages of colorectal cancer or who previously had polyps removed.

NSAIDs can cause serious or even life-threatening bleeding from stomach irritation, which may outweigh the benefits of these medicines for the general public. For this reason, experts do not recommend NSAIDs as a cancer prevention strategy for people at average risk of having colorectal cancer.

The value of NSAIDs for people with an increased colorectal cancer risk is being actively studied. Celecoxib (Celebrex) has been approved by the U.S. Food and Drug Administration (FDA) for reducing polyp formation in people with familial adenomatous polyposis (FAP). Whereas this drug may cause less bleeding in the stomach than other NSAIDs, it may increase the risk of heart attacks and strokes. A similar drug, rofecoxib (Vioxx), was taken off the market because people who took it had an increased number of heart attacks and strokes.

Because aspirin or other NSAIDs can have serious **side effects,** check with your doctor before starting to take any of them on a regular basis.

Hormone Replacement Therapy

Hormone replacement therapy (HRT) consisting of estrogen and progesterone may reduce the risk of developing colorectal cancer in postmenopausal women, although cancer found in women on HRT may be at a more advanced stage.

HRT also lowers the risk of osteoporosis. It can also increase some risks, including the risk of heart disease, blood clots, and breast and uterine cancers. The decision whether to use HRT should be based on a careful discussion of the possible benefits and risks with your doctor.

Can Colorectal Polyps and Cancer Be Found Early?

This section describes tests that are used to look for colorectal polyps and cancer. The current American Cancer Society screening guidelines for colorectal cancer are also discussed.

Types of Colorectal Cancer Screening Tests

Screening is the process of looking for cancer in people who have no symptoms of the disease. Several different tests can be used to screen for colorectal cancer. These tests can be divided into 2 broad groups:

Tests that can find both colorectal polyps and cancer

These tests look at the structure of the colon itself to find any abnormal areas. This is done either with a scope inserted into the rectum or with special imaging tests. Polyps found before they turn cancerous can be removed, so these tests may prevent colorectal cancer. Because of this, they are preferred if they are available and you are willing to have them.

Tests that mainly find cancer

These involve testing the stool (feces) for signs that cancer may be present. These tests are less invasive and easier to have done, but they are less likely to detect polyps.

These tests (as well as others) can also be used when people have symptoms of colorectal cancer and other digestive diseases.

Screening Tests That Can Find Both Colorectal Polyps and Cancer

Flexible sigmoidoscopy

During flexible sigmoidoscopy, the doctor looks at part of the colon and rectum with a sigmoidoscope—a flexible, lighted tube about the thickness of a finger with a small video camera on the end. It is inserted through the rectum into the lower part of the colon. Images from the scope are viewed on a display monitor.

Using the sigmoidoscope, your doctor can view the inside of the rectum and part of the colon to detect (and possibly remove) any abnormality.

Because the sigmoidoscope is only 60 cm (about 2 feet) long, the doctor is able to see the entire rectum but less than half of the colon with this procedure.

Before the test

You will need to have a bowel preparation to clean out your lower colon. The colon and rectum must be empty and clean so your doctor can view the lining of the sigmoid colon and rectum. Your doctor will give you specific instructions to follow. You may be asked to follow a special diet (such as drinking only clear liquids) for a day before the exam. You may also be asked to use an **enema** or take a strong **laxative** to clean out your colon before the exam.

During the test

A sigmoidoscopy usually takes 10 to 20 minutes. Most people do not need to be sedated for this test, but this may be an option you can discuss with your doctor. Whereas sedation may alleviate discomfort during the test, it requires having someone with you to take you home after the test. You will likely be placed on a table on your left side with your knees positioned near your chest.

Your doctor should do a digital rectal exam (DRE) before inserting the sigmoidoscope. The sigmoidoscope is lubricated so it is easy to insert into the rectum. The scope may feel cool going in. The sigmoidoscope may stretch the wall of the colon, which may cause muscle spasms or lower abdominal pain. Air will be placed into the sigmoid colon through the sigmoidoscope so the doctor can better view the colon. During the procedure, you might feel pressure and slight cramping in your lower abdomen. To ease discomfort and the urge to have a bowel movement, it helps to breathe deeply and slowly through your mouth. You will feel better after the test once the air leaves your colon.

If a small polyp is found during the test, your doctor may remove it with a small instrument passed through the scope. The polyp will be sent to a laboratory to be looked at by a pathologist. If a precancerous polyp or colorectal cancer is found during the test, you will need to have a colonoscopy at a later date to look for polyps or cancer in the rest of the colon.

Possible complications and side effects

Sigmoidoscopy may be uncomfortable because of the air put into the colon, but it should not be painful. Be sure to let your doctor know if you feel pain during the procedure. You may see a small amount of blood in your first bowel movement after the test. Significant bleeding and puncture of the colon are possible complications, but they are uncommon.

Colonoscopy

During a colonoscopy, the doctor looks at the entire length of the colon and rectum with a colonoscope, which is basically a longer version of a sigmoidoscope. It is inserted through the rectum into the colon. The colonoscope has a video camera on the end that is connected to a display monitor so the doctor can see and closely examine the inside of the colon. Special instruments can be passed through the colonoscope to remove any suspicious looking areas such as polyps, if needed. Colonoscopy may be done in a hospital outpatient department, in a clinic, or in a doctor's office.

Before the test

The colon and rectum must be empty and clean so your doctor can view their inner linings during the test. You will need to take laxatives (liquids, pills, or both) the day before the test and possibly an enema that morning. Your doctor will give you specific instructions. It is important to read these carefully a few days ahead of time, since you may need to shop for special supplies and get laxatives from a pharmacy. If you are not sure about any part of the instructions, call the doctor's office and go over them step-by-step with the nurse. Many people consider the bowel preparation to be the most unpleasant part of the test, as it usually requires you to be in the bathroom quite a bit.

You may be given other instructions as well. For example, your doctor may instruct that you drink only clear liquids (water, apple juice, or cranberry juice, and any gelatin except red or purple) for a day or two before the exam. Plain tea or coffee with sugar is usually okay, but no milk or creamer is allowed. Clear broth, ginger ale, and most soft drinks or sports drinks are usually allowed unless they have red or purple food colorings, which can discolor the colon.

You will likely also be told not to eat or drink anything after midnight the night before your test.

If you normally take prescription medicines in the mornings, talk with your doctor or nurse beforehand about how to manage them for the day.

You may need to arrange for someone to drive you home from the test because the sedative used during the test can affect your ability to drive. Depending on the medicines that are used, some doctors require that someone drive you home.

During the test

The test itself usually takes about 30 minutes, although it may take longer if a polyp is found and removed. Before the colonoscopy begins, you will be given a sedating medicine through your vein to make you feel comfortable and sleepy during the procedure. You will probably be awake, but you may not be aware of what is going on and may not remember the procedure afterward. Most people will be fully awake by the time they get home from the test.

During the procedure, you will be placed on your side with your knees flexed and a drape will cover you. Your blood pressure, heart rate, and breathing rate will be monitored during and after the test.

Your doctor should do a digital rectal exam (DRE) before inserting the colonoscope. The colonoscope is lubricated so it can be easily inserted into the rectum. Once in the rectum, the colonoscope is passed through the transverse colon and into the ascending colon. You may feel an urge to have a bowel movement when the colonoscope is inserted or pushed further up the colon. To ease any discomfort, it may help to breathe deeply and slowly through your mouth. The colonoscope will deliver air into the colon so that it is easier to see the lining of the colon and use the instruments to perform the test. Suction will be used to remove any blood or liquid stools.

If any small polyps are found, the doctor will probably remove them. Some small polyps may eventually become cancerous. To remove a polyp, the doctor passes a wire loop through the colonoscope to cut the polyp from the wall of the colon with an electrical current. The polyp can then be sent to a laboratory to be checked under a microscope to see if it has any areas that have changed into cancer.

If your doctor sees a large polyp or anything else abnormal, a biopsy may be done. For this procedure, a small piece of tissue is taken out through the colonoscope. The tissue is looked at under a microscope to determine whether it is cancer, a benign (noncancerous) growth, or a result of inflammation.

Possible side effects and complications

The bowel preparation before the test can be unpleasant. The test itself may be uncomfortable, but the sedative usually prevents this discomfort, and most people feel normal once the effects of the sedative wear off. Some people may have gas pains or cramping for awhile after the test.

In some cases, people may have low blood pressure or changes in heart rhythms due to the sedation during the test, although these are rarely serious.

If a polyp is removed or a biopsy is done during the colonoscopy, you may notice some blood in your stool for a day or two after the test. Significant bleeding is slightly more likely with colonoscopy than with sigmoidoscopy, but it is still uncommon. In rare cases, continued bleeding might require treatment.

Although colonoscopy is a safe procedure, on rare occasions the colonoscope can puncture the wall of the colon or rectum. This is called a perforation. It can be a serious complication and at times requires surgical repair. Talk to your doctor about the risk of this complication.

Double-contrast barium enema

A double-contrast barium enema (DCBE) is also called an *air-contrast barium enema* or a *barium enema with air contrast.* It is basically a type of x-ray. Barium sulfate, which is a chalky liquid, and air are used to outline the inner part of the colon and rectum to look for abnormal areas on x-rays. If suspicious areas are seen on this test, a colonoscopy will be needed to explore them further.

Before the test

As with colonoscopy, it is very important that the colon and rectum are empty and clean so your doctor can view them during the test. Your doctor will give you specific instructions on preparing for the test. Be sure to follow them. For example, you may be asked to take laxatives the night before or use an enema the morning of the exam. You will likely be asked to follow a diet of clear liquids for a day or two before the procedure. You may also be told to avoid eating or drinking dairy products the day before the test and not to eat or drink anything after midnight on the night before the procedure. Many people consider the bowel preparation to be the most unpleasant part of the test, as it usually requires you to be in the bathroom quite a bit.

During the test

The procedure takes about 30 to 45 minutes to perform, and it does not require sedation. For this test, you lie on a table on your side in an x-ray room. A small, flexible tube is inserted into the rectum, and barium sulfate is used to partially fill and open up the colon. When the colon is about half-full of barium, your body is turned on the x-ray table so the barium spreads throughout the colon. Then air is pumped into the colon through the same tube to make it expand. This may cause some discomfort, and you may feel the urge to have a bowel movement.

X-ray pictures of the lining of your colon are then taken, allowing the doctor to identify any polyps or cancer. You may be asked to change positions so that different views of the colon and rectum can be seen on the x-rays.

If polyps or other suspicious areas are seen on this test, a colonoscopy will likely be needed to remove them or to explore them more fully.

Possible side effects and complications

You may have bloating or cramping after the test and will likely feel the need to empty your bowels almost immediately after the test is done. The barium can cause constipation for a few days, and your stool may appear grey or white until the barium leaves the body. There is a very small risk that inflating the colon with air could injure or puncture the colon, but the risk for injury with barium enema is much lower than that associated with colonoscopy.

CT colonography (virtual colonoscopy)

CT colonography, commonly called a virtual colonoscopy, is an advanced type of computed tomography (also called CT scan or CAT scan) of the colon and rectum. A CT scan is an x-ray test that produces detailed cross-sectional images of your body. Instead of taking one picture, like a regular x-ray, a CT scanner takes many pictures as it rotates around you while you lie on a table. A computer then combines these pictures into images of slices of the part of your body being studied. CT colonography involves the use of special computer programs to create both 2-dimensional x-ray pictures and a 3-dimensional "fly-through" view of the inside of the colon and rectum, which allows the doctor to look for polyps or cancer.

This test may be especially useful for some people who cannot have or do not want to have more invasive tests such as colonoscopy. It can be done fairly quickly and does not require sedation.

Whereas this test is not invasive, like colonoscopy, it still requires the same type of bowel preparation. If polyps or other suspicious areas are seen on this test, a colonoscopy will likely be needed to remove them or to explore them more fully.

Before the test

It is important that the colon and rectum are emptied before CT colonography to provide the best images. Because of this, the preparation for this test is similar to that for a double-contrast barium enema or colonoscopy. You will likely be told to follow a diet of clear liquids for a day or two before the test. You will also be given instructions for taking strong laxatives and/or enemas the night before or the morning of the exam. This will likely require you to be in the bathroom quite a bit.

During the test

CT colonography is done in a special room with a CT scanner and takes about 10 minutes. You may be asked to drink a contrast solution before the test to help "tag" any remaining stool in the colon or rectum, which helps the doctor when looking at the test images. You will be asked to lie on a thin table that is part of the CT scanner, and you will have a small, flexible tube inserted into your rectum. Air is pumped through the tube into the colon to expand it to provide better images. The table then slides into the CT scanner, and you will be asked to hold your breath while the scan takes place. You will likely have 2 scans: one while you are lying on your back and one while you are on your stomach. Each scan typically takes only about 10 to 15 seconds.

Possible side effects and complications

There are usually very few side effects after CT colonography. You may feel bloated or have cramps due to the air in the colon, but this should go away once the air passes from the body. There is a very small risk that inflating the colon with air could injure or puncture the colon, but the risk for injury with CT colonography is much lower than that associated with colonoscopy.

Screening Tests That Mainly Find Colorectal Cancer

Tests used to examine the stool to look for signs of cancer are believed to be easier because they are not invasive and can often be done at home. They are not as effective for detecting polyps as the tests described in the previous section, and a positive result on one of these screening tests will likely require a more invasive test such as colonoscopy.

Fecal occult blood test

The fecal occult blood test (FOBT) is used to find occult (hidden) blood in feces. The idea behind this test is that blood vessels at the surface of larger colorectal polyps or cancerous tumors are often fragile and easily damaged by the passage of feces. The damaged vessels usually release a small amount of blood into the feces, but only rarely is there enough bleeding to be noticeable in the stool.

The FOBT detects blood in the stool through a chemical reaction but does not reveal whether the blood is from the colon or from other portions of the digestive tract (such as the stomach). Therefore, if the test detects blood, a colonoscopy is needed to see whether there is a cancer, polyp, or other cause of bleeding such as ulcers, hemorrhoids, diverticulosis (tiny pouches that form at weak spots in the colon wall), or inflammatory bowel disease (colitis).

The FOBT is a take-home kit that is used in the privacy of your own home. *An FOBT done during a digital rectal exam in the doctor's office is not sufficient for screening.* In order to be beneficial, the test must be repeated every year.

If you are taking the FOBT, you will receive a kit with instructions from the doctor's office or clinic. The kit will explain how to take a stool or feces sample at home (usually specimens from 3 consecutive bowel movements that are smeared onto small squares of paper). The kit should then be returned to the doctor's office or medical laboratory (usually within 2 weeks) for testing. See below for more details.

Before the test

Some foods or drugs can affect the test, so your doctor may suggest that you avoid the following before this test:

- nonsteroidal anti-inflammatory drugs (NSAIDs), such as ibuprofen (Advil or Motrin), naproxen (Aleve), or aspirin (more

than 1 adult aspirin per day). Avoid these
for 7 days before testing—they can cause
bleeding, which can lead to a false-positive
result. Acetaminophen (Tylenol) can be
taken as needed.

- vitamin C in excess of 250 mg daily
  from either supplements or citrus fruits
  and juices. Avoid these for 3 days before
  testing—they can affect the chemicals in
  the test and cause a false-negative result.
- red meats (beef, lamb, or liver). Avoid red
  meat for 3 days before testing—components of blood in the meat may cause the
  test to show positive.

Some people who are given the test never do it or
do not give it to their doctor because they worry
that something they ate may interfere with the test.
For this reason, many doctors tell their patients it
is not essential to follow any restrictions in their
diet. The most important thing is to get the test
done. People should try to avoid taking aspirin
or related drugs for minor aches. If you take these
medicines daily for heart problems or other conditions, do not stop them for this test without
approval from your doctor.

Collecting the samples

Have all of your supplies ready and in one place.
Supplies will include a test kit, test cards, either a
brush or wooden applicator, and a mailing envelope. The kit will give you detailed instructions
on how to collect the specimen. The instructions

below can be used as a guide, but your kit instructions might be a little different. Always follow the instructions included with your kit.

- You will need to collect a sample from your bowel movement. You can place a sheet of plastic wrap across the toilet bowl to catch the stool, or you can use a dry container to collect the stool. Do not let the stool specimen mix with urine. After you obtain a sample, you can flush the remaining stool down the toilet.
- Use a wooden applicator or a brush to smear a thin film of the stool sample onto one of the slots in the test card or slide.
- Next, collect a specimen from a different area of the same bowel movement and smear a thin film of the sample onto the other slot in the test card or slide.
- Close the slots and put your name and the date on the test kit. Store the kit overnight in a paper envelope to allow it time to dry.
- Repeat the test on your next 2 bowel movements if instructed. Most tests require collecting more than one sample from different bowel movements. This improves the accuracy of the test because many types of cancer bleed intermittently and blood may not be present in every stool sample.
- Place the test kit in the mailing envelope provided and return it to your doctor or laboratory as soon as possible (but within 14 days of taking the first sample).

If this test finds blood, a colonoscopy will be needed to look for the source. It is not sufficient to repeat the FOBT or follow up with other types of tests.

Fecal immunochemical test

The **fecal immunochemical test (FIT)**, also called an immunochemical fecal occult blood test (iFOBT), is a newer kind of test that also detects hidden blood in the stool. This test reacts to part of the **hemoglobin** molecule, which is found on red blood cells.

The FIT is done essentially the same way as the FOBT, but some people may find it easier to use because there are no drug or dietary restrictions (vitamins or foods do not affect the FIT) and sample collection may take less effort. This test is also less likely to react to bleeding from the upper digestive tract, such as the stomach.

As with the FOBT, the FIT may not detect a tumor that is not bleeding, so multiple stool samples should be tested. If the results are positive for hidden blood, a colonoscopy is required to investigate further. In order to be beneficial, the test must be repeated every year.

Collecting the samples

Have all of your supplies ready and in one place. Supplies will include a test kit, test cards, long brushes, waste bags, and a mailing envelope. The kit will give you detailed instructions on how to collect the specimen. The instructions below can be used as a guide, but your kit instructions might be a little different. Always follow the instructions included with your kit.

- Flush the toilet before your bowel movement. After you go to the bathroom, place used toilet paper in the waste bag included with the kit, not in the toilet.
- Brush the surface of the stool with one of the brushes, then dip the brush in the toilet water. Dab the end of the brush onto one of the slots in the test card or slide.
- Close the slot and put your name and the date on the test kit.
- Repeat the test on your next bowel movement if instructed. Most tests require that you collect samples from more than one bowel movement. Multiple samples improves the accuracy of the test because many types of cancer bleed intermittently and blood may not be present in every stool sample.
- Place the test kit in the mailing envelope provided and return it to your doctor or laboratory as soon as possible (but within 14 days of taking the first sample).

Stool DNA tests

Instead of looking for blood in the stool, the **stool DNA test** (sDNA test) looks for certain abnormal sections of DNA from cancer or polyp cells. Colorectal cancer cells often contain DNA mutations in certain genes such as APC, K-ras, and **p53**. Cells from colorectal cancer or polyps with these mutations are often shed into the stool, where tests may be able to detect them.

The stool DNA test is a newer test, and it is not yet clear how frequently it should be performed. This test is also much more expensive than other forms of stool testing. It is not invasive and does not require any special preparation. As with other stool tests, if the results are positive, a colonoscopy is required to investigate further.

People having this test will receive a kit with detailed instructions from their doctor's office or clinic on how to collect the specimen. Always follow the instructions included with your kit.

This test requires an entire stool sample. It is obtained by using a special container, which is placed in a bracket that stretches across the seat of the toilet. You have your bowel movement while sitting on the toilet, making sure it goes into the container. You then place the container and an ice pack in a shipping box and close and label the box. The specimen must be shipped to the laboratory within 24 hours of collection of the sample.

Pros and Cons of Various Screening Tests

Test	Pros	Cons
Flexible sigmoidoscopy	Fairly quick and safe Minimal bowel preparation Sedation usually not required Does not require a specialist Done every 5 years	Views only about a third of the colon Can't remove all polyps May cause some discomfort Done in a doctor's office, clinic, or hospital Very small risk of bleeding, infection, or bowel tear Colonoscopy needed if abnormal results
Colonoscopy	Can usually view entire colon Can biopsy and remove polyps Done every 10 years Can diagnose other diseases	Can miss small polyps Full bowel preparation needed More expensive on a one-time basis than other forms of testing Sedation of some kind is usually needed You will need someone to drive you home You may miss a day of work Small risk of bleeding, bowel tears, or infection
Double-contrast barium enema (DCBE)	Can usually view entire colon Relatively safe Done every 5 years No sedation needed	Can miss small polyps Full bowel preparation needed Some false-positive test results Cannot remove polyps during testing Colonoscopy still needed if results are abnormal

Test	Pros	Cons
CT colonography (virtual colonoscopy)	Fairly quick and safe Can usually view entire colon Done every 5 years No sedation needed	Can miss small polyps Full bowel preparation needed Some false-positive test results Cannot remove polyps during testing Colonoscopy still needed if results are abnormal Still fairly new, so possible insurance issues
Fecal occult blood test (FOBT)	No direct risk to the colon No bowel preparation Sampling done at home Inexpensive	Can miss many polyps and some cancers Can produce false-positive test results May have pretest dietary limitations Should be done annually Colonoscopy still needed if abnormal results
Fecal immunochemical test (FIT)	No direct risk to the colon No bowel preparation No pretest dietary restrictions Sampling done at home Fairly inexpensive	Can miss many polyps and some cancers Can produce false-positive test results Should be done annually Colonoscopy still needed if abnormal results
Stool DNA (sDNA) test	No direct risk to the colon No bowel preparation No pretest dietary restrictions Sampling done at home	Can miss many polyps and some cancers Can produce false-positive test results More expensive than other stool tests Still a fairly new test Not clear how often it should be done Colonoscopy still needed if results are abnormal

American Cancer Society Recommendations for Colorectal Cancer Early Detection

People at Average Risk

The American Cancer Society believes that preventing colorectal cancer—not just finding it early—should be a major reason for getting tested. Finding and removing polyps keeps some people from getting colorectal cancer. Flexible sigmoidoscopy, colonoscopy, double-contrast barium enemas, and CT colonography—the tests that have the best chance of finding both polyps and cancer—are preferred over the 3 types of stool tests if these tests are available to you and you are willing to have them.

Beginning at age 50, both men and women at *average risk* for developing colorectal cancer should use *one* of the screening tests below:

Tests that find polyps and cancer
- flexible sigmoidoscopy every 5 years*
- colonoscopy every 10 years
- double-contrast barium enema every 5 years*
- CT colonography (virtual colonoscopy) every 5 years*

Tests that mainly find cancer
- fecal occult blood test (FOBT) every year*[†]

---

* Colonoscopy should be done if test results are positive.
[†] For FOBT used as a screening test, the take-home multiple sample method should be used. An FOBT done during a digital rectal exam in the doctor's office is not adequate for screening.

- **fecal immunochemical test (FIT) every year***
- **stool DNA test (sDNA), interval uncertain***

In a digital rectal examination (DRE), a doctor examines your rectum with a lubricated, gloved finger. Although a DRE is often included as part of a routine physical exam, it is not recommended as a stand-alone test for colorectal cancer. This simple test, which is not usually painful, can detect masses in the anal canal or lower rectum. By itself, however, it is not a very sensitive test for detecting colorectal cancer because of its limited reach.

Doctors often find a small amount of stool when doing a DRE. However, simply checking stool obtained in this fashion for evidence of bleeding with a fecal occult blood test or fecal immunochemical test is not an acceptable method of screening for colorectal cancer. Research has shown that this type of stool examination will miss more than 90% of colon abnormalities, including most types of cancer.

People at Increased or High Risk

If you are at an increased risk for colorectal cancer, you should begin colorectal cancer screening earlier and/or be screened more often than those at average risk. The following conditions place you at higher than average risk:

---

* Colonoscopy should be done if test results are positive.

- a personal history of colorectal cancer or adenomatous polyps
- a personal history of inflammatory bowel disease (ulcerative colitis or Crohn's disease)
- a strong family history of colorectal cancer or polyps (see pages 13–14)
- a known family history of hereditary colorectal cancer syndromes such as familial adenomatous polyposis (FAP) or hereditary nonpolyposis colon cancer (HNPCC)

The table on pages 54–57 suggests screening guidelines for those with *increased or high risk* of colorectal cancer based on specific risk factors. Some people may have more than one risk factor. Refer to the table, and discuss these recommendations with your doctor. Based on your individual situation and any risk factors you may have, your doctor can suggest the best screening option for you, as well as any changes in the screening schedule based on your individual risk.

American Cancer Society Guidelines on Screening and Surveillance for the Early Detection of Colorectal Adenomas and Cancer in People at Increased Risk or High Risk

INCREASED RISK: Patients with a History of Polyps on Prior Colonoscopy

Risk Category	Age to Begin Screening	Recommended Test(s)	Comment
People with small rectal hyperplastic polyps	Same as if at average risk	Colonoscopy, or other screening options at same intervals as for those at average risk	Those with hyperplastic polyposis syndrome are at increased risk for adenomatous polyps and cancer and should have more intensive follow-up.
People with 1 or 2 small (less than 1 cm) tubular adenomas with low-grade dysplasia	5 to 10 years after the polyps are removed	Colonoscopy	Time between tests should be based on other factors such as prior colonoscopy findings, family history, and patient and doctor preferences.
People with 3 to 10 adenomas, or a large (≥1 cm) adenoma, or any adenomas with high-grade dysplasia or villous features	3 years after the polyps are removed	Colonoscopy	Adenomas must have been completely removed. If colonoscopy is normal or shows only 1 or 2 small tubular adenomas with low-grade dysplasia, future colonoscopies can be done every 5 years.
People with >10 adenomas on a single exam	Within 3 years after the polyps are removed	Colonoscopy	Doctor should consider possibility of genetic syndrome (such as FAP or HNPCC).

FAP, familial adenomatous polyposis; HNPCC, hereditary nonpolyposis colon cancer.

Risk Category	Age to Begin Screening	Recommended Test(s)	Comment
People with sessile adenomas that are removed in pieces	2 to 6 months after adenoma removal	Colonoscopy	If entire adenoma has been removed, further testing should be based on doctor's judgment.

INCREASED RISK: Patients with Colorectal Cancer

Risk Category	Age to Begin Screening	Recommended Test(s)	Comment
People diagnosed with colon or rectal cancer	At time of colorectal surgery, or can be 3 to 6 months later if person does not have metastatic tumors that cannot be removed during surgery.	Colonoscopy to view entire colon and remove all polyps	If the tumor presses on the colon/rectum and prevents colonoscopy, CT colonography (with IV contrast) or DCBE may be done to look at the rest of the colon.
People who have had colon or rectal cancer removed by surgery	Within 1 year after cancer resection (or 1 year after colonoscopy to make sure the rest of the colon/rectum was clear)	Colonoscopy	If normal, repeat exam in 3 years. If normal then, repeat exam every 5 years. Time between tests may be shorter if polyps are found or there is reason to suspect HNPCC. After low anterior resection for rectal cancer, rectal exams may be done every 3 to 6 months for the first 2 to 3 years to look for signs of recurrence.

CT colonography (CT = computed tomography); IV, intravenous; DCBE, double-contrast barium enema.

INCREASED RISK: Patients with a Family History

Risk Category	Age to Begin Screening	Recommended Test(s)	Comment
Colorectal cancer or adenomatous polyps in any first-degree relative before age 60, or in 2 or more first-degree relatives at any age (if not a hereditary syndrome)	Age 40, or 10 years before the youngest case in the immediate family, whichever is earlier	Colonoscopy	Every 5 years
Colorectal cancer or adenomatous polyps in any first-degree relative aged 60 or higher, or in at least 2 second-degree relatives at any age	Age 40	Colonoscopy	Every 10 years

HIGH RISK

Risk Category	Age to Begin Screening	Recommended Test(s)	Comment
FAP diagnosed by genetic testing, or suspected FAP without genetic testing	Age 10 to 12	Yearly flexible sigmoidoscopy to look for signs of FAP; counseling to consider genetic testing if it hasn't been done	If genetic test is positive, removal of colon (colectomy) should be considered.
Hereditary nonpolyposis colon cancer (HNPCC), or at increased risk of HNPCC based on family history without genetic testing	Age 20 to 25 years, or 10 years before the youngest case in the immediate family	Colonoscopy every 1 to 2 years; counseling to consider genetic testing if it hasn't been done	Genetic testing should be offered to first-degree relatives of people found to have HNPCC mutations by genetic tests. It should also be offered if 1 of the first 3 of the Bethesda Guidelines is met. *
Inflammatory bowel disease -Chronic ulcerative colitis -Crohn's disease	Cancer risk begins to be significant 8 years after the onset of pancolitis (involvement of entire large intestine), or 12 to 15 years after the onset of left-sided colitis	Colonoscopy every 1 to 2 years, with biopsies for dysplasia	These people are best referred to a center with experience in the surveillance and management of inflammatory bowel disease.

*The Bethesda Guidelines can be found on pages 25–26.
FAP, familial adenomatous polyposis; HPNCC, hereditary nonpolyposis colon cancer.

Insurance Coverage for Colorectal Cancer Screening

Despite the availability of effective colorectal cancer screening tests, not enough people have them. The reasons for this could include lack of public and health professional awareness of screening tools, financial barriers, and inadequate health insurance coverage and/or benefits.

Laws regarding insurance coverage for colorectal cancer screening tests vary by state. The same is true of state Medicaid programs. For people with Medicare, coverage begins at age 50 for the most common colorectal cancer screening tests.

For more information on insurance coverage for colorectal cancer screening tests, contact the American Cancer Society at **800-ACS-2345** and ask for the document *Colorectal Cancer: Early Detection* or visit our Web site at **www.cancer.org**.

Diagnosis and Staging

How Is Colorectal Cancer Diagnosed?

Whereas colorectal cancer is often found after symptoms appear, most people with early colon or rectal cancer have no symptoms of the disease. Symptoms usually appear only with more advanced disease. This is why getting the recommended screening tests (described in the previous chapter) before symptoms develop is so important.

If your doctor finds something suspicious during a screening exam, or if you have any of the symptoms of colorectal cancer described below, you will likely need to undergo a diagnostic workup.

Signs and Symptoms of Colorectal Cancer

If you have any of the following, you should check with your doctor for prompt **diagnosis** and treatment:

- a change in bowel habits, such as diarrhea, constipation, or narrowing of the stool, that lasts for more than a few days
- a feeling that you need to have a bowel movement that is not relieved by doing so

- rectal bleeding, dark stools, or blood in the stool (though stool will often look normal)
- cramping or abdominal pain
- weakness and fatigue

Most of these symptoms are more likely to be caused by conditions other than colorectal cancer, such as infection, hemorrhoids, or inflammatory bowel disease. Still, if you have any of these problems, it is important to see your doctor right away so the cause can be found and, if needed, treated. Your doctor may perform the following tests.

Medical History and Physical Examination

If you have any signs or symptoms that suggest you might have colorectal cancer, your doctor will want to take a complete medical history to check for symptoms and risk factors, including your family history.

As part of a physical examination, your doctor will carefully feel your abdomen for masses or enlarged organs and will also examine the rest of your body. Your doctor may also perform a digital rectal exam. During this test, the doctor inserts a lubricated, gloved finger into the rectum to feel for any abnormal areas.

Blood Tests

Your doctor may also order certain blood tests to help determine whether you have colorectal cancer.

Complete blood count

Your doctor may order a **complete blood count (CBC)** to see whether you have **anemia** (too few **red blood cells**). Some people with colorectal cancer become anemic because of prolonged bleeding from the tumor. You may also have a blood test of your liver function, because colorectal cancer can spread to the liver and cause abnormalities.

Tumor markers

Colorectal cancer sometimes produces substances such as **carcinoembryonic antigen (CEA)** and **CA 19-9**. These substances are released into the bloodstream. Blood tests for these "**tumor markers**" are used most often with other tests for follow-up of patients who already have been treated for colorectal cancer. They may provide early warning that a cancer has returned.

CEA and CA 19-9 are not used to find cancer in people who have never had cancer and appear to be healthy because the tests are not always accurate. Tumor marker levels can be normal in a person who has cancer and can be abnormal for reasons other than cancer. For example, higher levels may also be present in the blood of some people with ulcerative colitis, noncancerous tumors of the intestines, or some types of liver disease or chronic lung disease. Smoking can also raise CEA levels.

Tests to Detect Colorectal Polyps or Cancer

If symptoms or the results of the physical examination or blood tests suggest that colorectal cancer might be present, your doctor may recommend additional tests. These might include endoscopic tests such as sigmoidoscopy or colonoscopy or imaging tests such as a barium enema (commonly called a **lower GI series**), double-contrast barium enema, or CT colonography (virtual colonoscopy). Most of these tests are described in detail on pages 31–50.

Biopsy

Usually, if a suspected colorectal cancer is found by any diagnostic test, it is biopsied during a colonoscopy. In a biopsy, the doctor passes a special instrument through the scope to remove a small piece of tissue. The tissue is sent to the laboratory, where a pathologist, a doctor trained to diagnose cancer and other diseases in tissue samples, looks at the tissue under a microscope. Whereas other tests may suggest that colorectal cancer is present, a biopsy is the only way to determine this for certain.

Imaging Tests

Imaging tests use sound waves, x-rays, magnetic fields, or radioactive substances to create pictures of the inside of your body. Imaging tests may be done for a number of reasons, including to help find out whether a suspicious area might be cancerous, to learn how far cancer may have spread, and to help determine if treatment has been effective.

Computed tomography

A computed tomography scan (CT scan or CAT scan) is an x-ray test that produces detailed cross-sectional images of your body. Instead of taking one picture, like a regular x-ray, a CT scanner takes many pictures as it rotates around you while you lie on a table. A computer then combines these pictures into images of the part of your body being studied. Unlike a regular x-ray, a CT scan creates detailed images of the soft tissues in the body. This test can help tell if colon cancer has spread into your liver or other organs.

After the first set of pictures is taken, you may be asked to drink a contrast solution and/or receive an **intravenous (IV) line** through which a contrast dye is injected. This helps better outline structures in your body. A second set of pictures is then taken.

The contrast may cause some flushing (a feeling of warmth, especially in the face). Some people are allergic to the contrast solution and get hives. Rarely, more serious reactions like trouble breathing or low blood pressure can occur. Be sure to tell the doctor if you have ever had a reaction to any contrast material used for x-rays.

CT scans take longer than regular x-rays. You need to lie still on a table while they are being done. During the test, the table moves in and out of the scanner, a ring-shaped machine that completely surrounds the table. You might feel a bit confined by the ring you have to lie in while the pictures are being taken.

In recent years, **spiral CT** (also known as **helical CT**) has become available in many medical centers. This type of CT scan uses a faster machine. The scanner part of the machine rotates around the body continuously, allowing doctors to collect the images much more quickly than with standard CT. This lowers the chance of "blurred" images occurring as a result of motion caused by breathing. It also lowers the dose of radiation received during the test. The biggest advantage may be that it yields more detailed pictures and allows doctors to look at suspicious areas from different angles.

For spiral CT with *portography* (looking at the **portal vein**—the large vein leading into the liver from the intestine), contrast material is injected into veins that lead to the liver, to help find any areas where colorectal cancer has spread to the liver.

CT–guided needle biopsy

CT scans can also be used to precisely guide a biopsy needle into a suspected tumor or metastasis, called a **CT–guided needle biopsy.** For this procedure, the patient remains on the CT scanning table while a **radiologist** advances a biopsy needle through the skin and toward the location of the mass. CT scans are repeated until the doctors are confident that the needle is within the mass. A fine-needle biopsy sample (tiny fragment of tissue) or a core needle biopsy sample (a thin cylinder of tissue about ½-inch long and less than ⅛ inch in diameter) is then removed and looked at under a microscope.

CT colonography (virtual colonoscopy)

CT scans can also be used to perform a CT colonography or "virtual colonoscopy." This test requires the same type of bowel preparation as that used for colonoscopy. Before the scan is done, the colon is inflated with air so that it can be viewed more clearly; this stretches the colon and can cause some discomfort.

Spiral CT of the abdomen is then done. The thin pictures it obtains can be combined to create 2- and 3-dimensional views of the colon and rectum. If abnormalities are detected, a follow-up colonoscopy will be needed to take tissue samples of the abnormal areas.

Ultrasound

Ultrasound involves the use of sound waves and their echoes to produce a picture of internal organs or masses. A small microphone-like instrument called a transducer emits sound waves and picks up the echoes as they bounce off body tissues. The echoes are converted by a computer into a black and white image that is displayed on a computer screen. This test is painless and does not expose you to radiation.

Abdominal ultrasound can be used to look for tumors in your liver, gallbladder, pancreas, or even inside your abdomen, although it cannot look for tumors of the colon. When you have an abdominal ultrasound exam, you simply lie on a table and a technician moves the transducer over the skin overlying the part of your body being examined. Usually, the skin is first lubricated with gel.

Two special types of ultrasound examinations can be used to evaluate people with colon and rectal cancer.

Endorectal ultrasound uses a special transducer that can be inserted directly into the rectum. This test is used to see how far through the wall of the rectum a cancer may have penetrated and whether it has spread to nearby organs or tissues such as lymph nodes.

Intraoperative ultrasound is done after the surgeon has opened the abdominal cavity. The transducer can be placed against the surface of the liver, making this test very useful in detecting metastases of colorectal cancer to the liver.

Magnetic resonance imaging

Like CT scans, magnetic resonance imaging (MRI) scans provide detailed images of soft tissues in the body. MRI scans use radio waves and strong magnets instead of x-rays. The energy from the radio waves is absorbed and then released in a pattern formed by the type of body tissue and by certain diseases. A computer translates the pattern into a very detailed image of parts of the body. A contrast material called gadolinium is often injected into a vein before the scan to better see details.

MRI scans cause a little more discomfort than do CT scans. First, MRI scans take longer—often up to an hour. Second, you have to lie inside a narrow tube, which is confining and can upset people with claustrophobia (a fear of enclosed spaces). Newer, "open" MRI machines are sometimes available and can be helpful for people with this concern. The machine also makes buzzing and thumping noises that you may find disturbing. Some centers provide headphones with music to block this out.

MRI scans are sometimes useful in looking at abnormal areas in the liver that might represent cancer spread. They can also help determine the extent of rectal cancer. To improve the accuracy of the test, some doctors use **endorectal MRI.** For this test the doctor places a probe, called an endorectal coil, inside the rectum. This must stay in place for 30 to 45 minutes and can be uncomfortable.

Chest x-ray

This test may be done after colorectal cancer has been diagnosed to determine whether the cancer has spread to the lungs.

Positron emission tomography

Positron emission tomography (PET) scans involve injecting a form of radioactive sugar (known as fluorodeoxyglucose, or FDG) into the blood. The amount of radioactivity used is very low. Because cancer cells in the body are growing rapidly, they absorb large amounts of the radioactive sugar. A special camera can then create a picture of areas of radioactivity in the body. The picture is not finely detailed like a CT or MRI scan, but it provides helpful information about your whole body.

PET scans are sometimes useful if your doctor thinks the cancer may have spread (or returned after treatment) but does not know where. PET scans can be used instead of several different x-rays because they scan your whole body.

Some newer machines are able to perform both a PET and CT scan at the same time (PET/CT scan). This allows the radiologist to compare areas of higher radioactivity on the PET with the appearance of that area on the CT.

Angiography

An **angiogram** is sometimes used to help plan surgery, especially for tumors in the liver. For this test, a doctor inserts a very thin tube (called a **catheter**) into an **artery,** usually on the inner thigh. The catheter is threaded through the artery until the tip is near the liver. Contrast dye is then injected and a series of x-rays is taken. The angiogram can show surgeons the location of blood vessels next to any tumors in the liver, so that tumors can be removed without causing a lot of bleeding.

How Is Colorectal Cancer Staged?

The **stage** describes the extent of the cancer in the body. It is based on how far the cancer has grown into the wall of the intestine, whether it has reached nearby structures, and whether it has spread to lymph nodes or distant organs. The stage of a cancer is one of the most important factors in determining prognosis and treatment.

Staging is the process of finding out how far a cancer has spread. It is based on the results of the physical examination, biopsies, and imaging tests described in the previous section, as well as the results of surgery.

There are actually 2 types of staging for colorectal cancer. The **clinical stage** is your doctor's best estimate of the extent of your disease, based on the results of the physical exam, biopsy, and any imaging tests you have had. If you have surgery, your doctors can also determine the **pathologic stage**, which is based on the same factors as the clinical stage, plus what is found during surgery and examination by microscope of any tissue removed during surgery. Because most patients with colorectal cancer have surgery, the pathologic stage is most often used when describing the extent of this cancer. Pathologic staging is more accurate than clinical staging, as it allows your doctor to get a firsthand impression of the extent of your disease.

AJCC (TNM) Staging System

A staging system is a standardized way to describe the extent of the cancer. The most commonly used staging system for colorectal cancer is the **American Joint Committee on Cancer staging system,** or **AJCC system,** sometimes also known as the TNM system. Two older systems, the **Dukes staging system** and the **Astler-Coller staging system,** are described briefly on page 74 for comparison.

The TNM system describes 3 key pieces of information:

- **T** describes how far the main tumor has grown into the wall of the intestine and whether it has grown into nearby areas.
- **N** describes the extent of spread to nearby lymph nodes. Lymph nodes are small bean-shaped collections of immune system cells that are important in fighting infections.
- **M** indicates whether the cancer has spread, or metastasized, to other organs of the body. The most common sites of spread for colorectal cancer are the liver and lungs, although it can spread anywhere.

Numbers or letters appear after T, N, and M to provide more detail. The numbers 0 through 4 indicate severity. The letter X means "cannot be assessed because the information is not available."

T categories for colorectal cancer

T categories of colorectal cancer describe the extent of spread through the layers that form the wall of the colon and rectum. These layers, from the inner to the outer, include—

- the inner lining (**mucosa**)
- a thin muscle layer (**muscularis mucosa**)
- the fibrous tissue beneath this muscle layer (**submucosa**)
- a thick muscle layer (**muscularis propria**) that contracts to force the contents of the intestines along
- the thin, outermost layers of connective tissue (**subserosa** and **serosa**) that cover most of the colon but not the rectum

Tx: No description of the tumor's extent is possible because of incomplete information.

Tis: The cancer is in the earliest stage. It involves only the mucosa. It has not grown beyond the muscularis mucosa (inner muscle layer). (Note: The abbreviation "is" means **in situ,** or in place.)

T1: The cancer has grown through the muscularis mucosa and extends into the submucosa.

T2: The cancer has grown through the submucosa and extends into the muscularis propria (outer muscle layer).

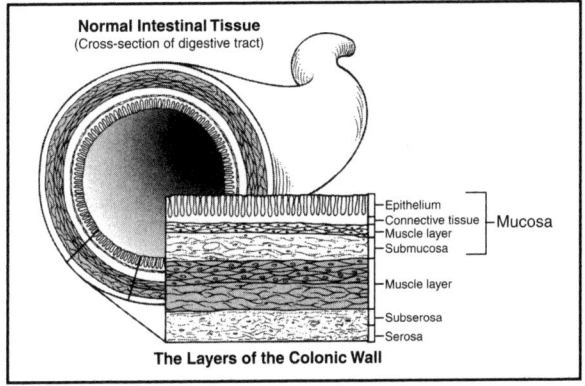

Normal Intestinal Tissue
(Cross-section of digestive tract)

Epithelium
Connective tissue — Mucosa
Muscle layer
Submucosa

Muscle layer

Subserosa

Serosa

The Layers of the Colonic Wall

T3: The cancer has grown through the muscularis propria and into the subserosa but not to any neighboring organs or tissues.

T4: The cancer has grown through the wall of the colon or rectum and into nearby tissues or organs.

N categories for colorectal cancer

N categories indicate whether the cancer has spread to nearby lymph nodes and, if so, how many lymph nodes are involved.

Nx: No description of lymph node involvement is possible because of incomplete information.

N0: No lymph node involvement is found.

N1: Cancer cells found in 1 to 3 nearby lymph nodes.

N2: Cancer cells found in 4 or more nearby lymph nodes.

M categories for colorectal cancer

M categories indicate whether the cancer has spread to distant organs, such as the liver, lungs, or distant lymph nodes.

Mx: No description of distant spread is possible because of incomplete information.

M0: No distant spread is seen.

M1: Distant spread is present.

Stage Grouping

Once a person's T, N, and M categories have been determined, usually after surgery, this information is combined in a process called *stage grouping*. The stage is expressed in Roman numerals from stage 0 (the least advanced) to stage IV (the most advanced). Some stages are subdivided with letters. The following guide illustrates how TNM categories are grouped together into stages:

Stage 0: Tis, N0, M0

The cancer is in the earliest stage. It has not grown beyond the inner layer (mucosa) of the colon or rectum. This stage is also known as **carcinoma in situ** and intramucosal carcinoma.

Stage I: T1, N0, M0, or T2, N0, M0

The cancer has grown through the muscularis mucosa into the submucosa (T1) *or* it may also have grown into the muscularis propria (T2). It has not spread to nearby lymph nodes or to distant sites.

Stage IIA: T3, N0, M0

The cancer has grown into the outermost layers of the colon or rectum but has not reached nearby organs. It has not yet spread to nearby lymph nodes or to distant sites.

Stage IIB: T4, N0, M0

The cancer has grown through the wall of the colon or rectum and into other nearby tissues or organs. It has not yet spread to nearby lymph nodes or to distant sites.

Stage IIIA: T1, N1, M0, or T2, N1, M0

The cancer has grown through the mucosa into the submucosa (T1) *or* it may also have grown into the muscularis propria (T2). It has spread to 1 to 3 nearby lymph nodes but not to distant sites.

Stage IIIB: T3, N1, M0, or T4, N1, M0

The cancer has grown into the outermost layers of the colon or rectum but has not reached nearby organs (T3) *or* the cancer has grown through the wall of the colon or rectum and into other nearby tissues or organs (T4). It has spread to 1 to 3 nearby lymph nodes but not to distant sites.

Stage IIIC: Any T, N2, M0

The cancer may or may not have grown through the wall of the colon or rectum, but it has spread to 4 or more nearby lymph nodes. It has not spread to distant sites.

Stage IV: Any T, Any N, M1

The cancer may or may not have grown through the wall of the colon or rectum, and it may or may not have spread to nearby lymph nodes. It has spread to distant sites such as the liver, lung, **peritoneum** (the membrane lining the abdominal cavity), or ovary.

Comparison of AJCC, Dukes, and Astler-Coller Stages

If your doctor refers to your stage in slightly different terms, he or she is likely referring to one of the other staging systems sometimes used for colorectal cancer, such as the Dukes system and Astler-Coller system. The table below can be used to find the matching AJCC/TNM stage. The Dukes and Astler-Coller staging systems often combine different AJCC stage groupings and are not as precise.

AJCC/TNM	Dukes	Astler-Coller
0	-	-
I	A	A, B1
IIA	B	B2
IIB	B	B3
IIIA	C	C1
IIIB	C	C2, C3
IIIC	C	C1, C2, C3
IV	-	D

If you have any questions about your stage, please ask your doctor to explain the extent of your disease.

Survival Rates for Colorectal Cancer

Survival rates are a way for doctors to discuss and compare the prognosis for patients based on the stage of the cancer or other traits. Please note these important points:

- The **5-year survival rate** refers to the percentage of patients who live *at least* 5 years after being diagnosed. Many of these patients live much longer than 5 years after diagnosis.

- While these numbers are among the most current we have available, they represent people who were first diagnosed and treated many years ago. Several improvements in treating colorectal cancer have been made since then, and the survival rates for people now being diagnosed with these types of cancer may be higher.

- Whereas survival statistics can sometimes be useful as a general guide, they may not accurately represent any one person's prognosis. A number of other factors, including other tumor characteristics and a person's age and general health, can also affect outlook. Your doctor is likely to be a good source to confirm whether these numbers may apply to you, as he or she will be familiar with your particular situation.

Survival Rates for Colon Cancer, by Stage

The numbers below come from a study of the National Cancer Institute's SEER database, which looked at nearly 120,000 people diagnosed with colon cancer between 1991 and 2000.

Stage	5-year Survival Rate
I	93%
IIA	85%
IIB	72%
IIIA	83%*
IIIB	64%
IIIC	44%
IV	8%

*In this study, survival was better for stage IIIA than for stage IIB. The reasons for this are not clear, and it is not known if this is still the case.

Relative Survival Rates for Rectal Cancer, by Stage

Accurate survival statistics for rectal cancer are a little harder to find, as it is a less common disease. The numbers below come from a study of the National Cancer Institute's SEER database, which looked at people diagnosed with rectal cancer between 1990 and 1999.

These numbers are *relative* survival rates. A standard 5-year survival rate refers to the percentage of patients who live at least 5 years after their cancer is diagnosed; it includes people with rectal cancer who may die of other causes, such as heart disease. The **relative five (5)-year survival rate** is adjusted for patients dying of other diseases, so they reflect the chances of not dying specifically of rectal cancer. As with standard survival rates, these rates are based on patients whose cancer was diagnosed and treated more than 5 years ago; improvements in treatment since then may result in a better outlook for recently diagnosed patients.

Stage	Relative 5-year Survival Rate
I	92%
II	73%
III	56%
IV	8%

Grade of Colorectal Cancer

One factor that can affect the outlook for survival is the **grade** of the cancer. Grade is a description of how closely the cancer resembles normal colorectal tissue when examined under a microscope.

The scale used for grading colorectal cancer goes from G1 (where the cancer looks much like normal colorectal tissue) to G4 (where the cancer looks very abnormal). The grades G2 and G3 fall somewhere in between. The grade is often simplified as either "low-grade" (G1 or G2) or "high-grade" (G3 or G4).

Most of the time, the outlook is not as favorable for high-grade cancer as it is for low-grade cancer. Doctors sometimes use this distinction to decide whether a patient should get extra treatment (**adjuvant therapy**) with chemotherapy after surgery (discussed in more detail on page 102).

Treatments

Your Medical Team

Your health care team will be made up of several people, each with different expertise to contribute to your care. One of your **cancer care team** members will take the lead in coordinating your care. Most colorectal cancer patients choose a medical oncologist to lead the team. It should be clear to all team members who is in charge, and that person should inform the others of your progress. This alphabetical list will acquaint you with the health care professionals you may encounter, depending on which treatment option and follow-up path you choose, and their areas of expertise:

Dietitian

A dietitian is specially trained to help you make healthy diet choices and maintain a healthy weight before, during, and after treatment. A registered dietitian (RD) has at least a bachelor's degree and has passed a national competency exam.

Gastroenterologist

Gastroenterologists are doctors who specialize in diseases of the digestive tract (also called the gastrointestinal tract). Most people with colorectal cancer receive their diagnosis from a gastroenterologist,

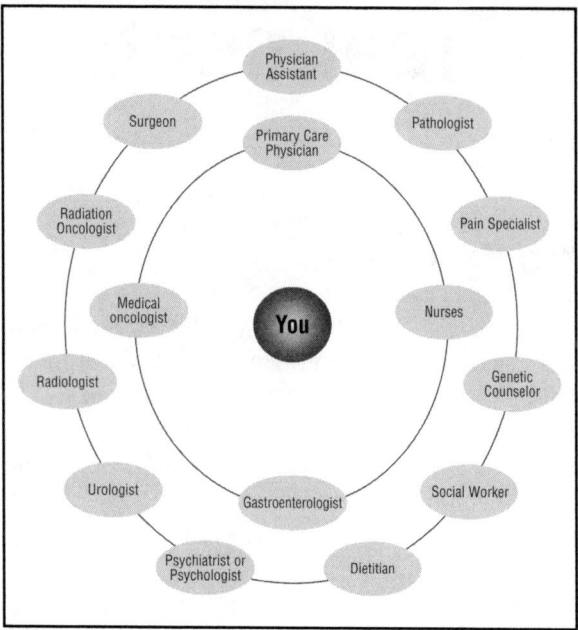

based on the results of their colonoscopy. After a diagnosis, the gastroenterologist will usually talk with your primary care physician to identify a surgeon and/or oncologist for you. He or she may arrange for tests to determine how far the cancer has spread and may also help you manage any changes in your bowel habits. The gastroenterologist will give you regular checkups after you finish your treatments. These checkups will include routine colonoscopies to make sure your colon and rectum remain cancer free.

Genetic Counselor

A genetic counselor is a health professional trained to help people through the process of genetic testing. A genetic counselor can explain the available tests to you, discuss the pros and cons, and address any concerns you might have. This counselor can arrange for genetic testing and then help interpret the test results. A certified genetic counselor has at least a master's degree and has passed both a general competency exam and a specialty genetic counseling exam.

Medical Oncologist

A medical oncologist (also sometimes called an oncologist) is a medical doctor you may see after diagnosis. The oncologist is a cancer expert who understands specific types of cancer, their treatments, and their causes. He or she may help cancer patients make decisions about a course of treatment and then manage all phases of cancer care. Oncologists most often become involved when you need chemotherapy, but can also prescribe hormonal therapy and other anticancer drugs.

Nurses

During your treatment you will be in contact with different types of nurses.

Registered nurse

A registered nurse has an associate or bachelor's degree in nursing and has passed a state licensing exam. He or she can monitor your condition, provide treatment, educate you about side effects, and help you adjust to cancer, both physically and emotionally.

Nurse practitioner

A nurse practitioner is a registered nurse with a master's degree or doctoral degree who can manage the care of patients with colorectal cancer and has additional training in primary care. He or she shares many tasks with your doctors, such as recording your medical history, conducting physical examinations, and doing follow-up care. In most states, a nurse practitioner can prescribe medications with a doctor's supervision.

Clinical nurse specialist

A clinical nurse specialist (CSN) is a nurse who has a master's degree in a specific area, such as oncology, psychiatry, or critical care nursing. The CSN often provides expertise to staff and may provide special services to patients, such as leading support groups and coordinating cancer care.

Oncology-certified nurse

An oncology-certified nurse is a clinical nurse who has demonstrated an in-depth knowledge of oncology care. He or she has passed a certification examination. Oncology-certified nurses are found in all areas of cancer practice.

Pain Specialist

Pain specialists are doctors, nurses, and pharmacists who are experts in managing pain. They can help you find pain control methods that are effective and allow you to maintain your quality of life.

Not all doctors and nurses are trained in pain care, so you may have to request a pain specialist if your pain relief needs are not being met.

Pathologist

A pathologist is a medical doctor specially trained in diagnosing disease based on examination of microscopic tissue and fluid samples. He or she will determine the classification (cell type) of your cancer, help determine the stage (extent) and grade (estimate of aggressiveness) of your cancer, and issue a pathology report so that you and your doctor can decide on treatment options.

Personal or Primary Care Physician

A personal physician may be a general doctor, internist, or family practice doctor. He or she is often the medical doctor you first saw when you noticed symptoms of illness. This general or family practice doctor may be a member of your medical team, but a specialist is most often a patient's cancer care team leader.

Physician Assistant

Physicians assistants (PAs) are health care professionals licensed to practice medicine with physician supervision. Physician assistants practice in the areas of primary care medicine (family medicine, internal medicine, pediatrics, and obstetrics and gynecology) as well as in surgery and the surgical subspecialties. Under the supervision of a doctor, they can diagnose and treat medical problems and, in most states, can also prescribe medications.

Psychologist or Psychiatrist

A psychologist is a licensed mental health professional who is often part of the cancer care team. He or she provides counseling on emotional and psychological issues. A psychologist may have specialized training and experience in treating people with cancer.

A psychiatrist is a medical doctor specializing in mental health and behavioral disorders. Psychiatrists provide counseling and can also prescribe medications.

Radiation Oncologist

A radiation oncologist is a medical doctor who specializes in treating cancer by using therapeutic radiation (high-energy x-rays or seeds). If you choose radiation, the radiation oncologist evaluates you frequently during the course of treatment and at intervals afterward. The radiation oncologist will usually work closely with your oncologist and will help you make decisions about radiation therapy options. A radiation oncologist is assisted by a radiation therapist during treatment and works with a radiation physicist, an expert who is trained in ensuring that you receive the correct dose of radiation treatment. The physicist is also assisted by a dosimetrist, a technician who helps plan and calculate the dosage, number, and length of your radiation treatments.

Radiologist

A radiologist is a medical doctor specializing in the use of imaging procedures (for example, diagnostic x-rays, ultrasound, magnetic resonance images, and bone scans) that produce pictures of internal body structures. He or she has special training in diagnosing cancer and other diseases and interpreting the results of imaging procedures. Your radiologist issues a radiology report describing the findings to your gastroenterologist, medical oncologist, or radiation oncologist. The radiology images and report may be used to aid in diagnosis; to help classify and determine the extent of your illness; to help locate tumors during procedures, surgery, and radiation treatment; or to look for the possible spread or recurrence of the cancer after treatment.

Social Worker

A social worker is a health specialist, usually with a master's degree, who is licensed or certified by the state in which he or she works. A social worker is an expert in coordinating and providing social services. He or she is trained to help you and your family deal with a range of emotional and practical challenges, such as finances, child care, emotional issues, family concerns and relationships, transportation, and problems with the health care system. If your social worker is trained in cancer-related problems, he or she can counsel you about your fears or concerns, help answer questions about diagnosis and treatment, and lead cancer support groups. You may communicate with your social worker during a hospital stay or on an outpatient basis.

Surgeon

Several different types of surgeons provide treatment for colorectal cancer. A general surgeon is trained to operate on all parts of the body, including the digestive tract. A surgical oncologist is a surgeon who has had advanced training in the surgical treatment of people with cancer. A colorectal surgeon is trained in general surgery but also has advanced training in the treatment of the colon and rectal problems including colorectal cancers. Cancer centers usually have one or more such individuals on their staff.

Although each type of surgeon has a different area of expertise, each plays the same role in treating people with colorectal cancer. If you require surgery as part of your treatment, the surgeon will perform the operation and then manage any side effects you might have. He or she will also issue a report to your other doctors to help determine the rest of your treatment plan.

Urologist

A urologist is a doctor who specializes in treating problems of the urinary tract in men and women and of the genital area in men. Colorectal cancer treatments occasionally cause side effects that require the expertise of a urologist. For example, radiation therapy can cause the bladder to become irritated, and some types of colorectal surgery can affect sexual function. If you experience these types of side effects, your doctors will probably consult with a urologist to address these conditions.

How Is Colorectal Cancer Treated?

This section describes the various types of treatments used for colon and rectal cancers, followed by a description of the treatment approaches most commonly used according to the stage of the cancer.

Making Treatment Decisions

The 4 main types of treatment for colon cancer and rectal cancer are **surgery, radiation therapy, chemotherapy,** and **targeted therapy.** Depending on the stage of the cancer, 2 or more of these types of treatment may be combined at the same time or used after one another.

After the cancer is found and staged, your cancer care team will discuss your treatment options with you. Take time and think about your possible choices. In choosing a treatment plan, one of the most important factors is the stage of the cancer. Other factors to consider include your overall health, the likely side effects of the treatment, and the probability of curing the disease, extending life, or relieving symptoms.

In considering your treatment options, it is often a good idea to seek a second opinion, if possible. A second opinion can provide you with more information and help you feel more confident about the treatment plan you have chosen. Your chances for having the best possible outcome are greatest if your medical team is experienced in treating colorectal cancer.

Surgery

The types of surgery used to treat cancer of the colon and rectum are slightly different and are described separately in the sections below.

Colon Surgery

Surgery is often the main treatment for earlier-stage colon cancer.

Colectomy

A **colectomy** (sometimes called a **hemicolectomy** or **segmental resection**) involves removing part of the colon as well as nearby lymph nodes.

Prior to surgery, you will need to make sure your bowels are completely empty. This is done with a bowel preparation, which may consist of laxatives and enemas. Just before the surgery, you will be given general **anesthesia,** which puts you into a deep sleep. During the surgery, your surgeon will make an incision in your abdomen. He or she will remove the cancer and a small segment of normal colon on either side of your cancer. Usually, about one-fourth to one-third of your colon is removed, but more or less tissue may be removed, depending on the exact size and location of your cancer. The remaining sections of your colon are then reattached. Nearby lymph nodes are removed at this time as well. Most experts believe that taking out as many nearby lymph nodes as possible is important, but at least 12 should be removed.

When you wake up after surgery, you will have some pain and will be given pain medicines for 2 or 3 days. For the first couple of days, you will be given intravenous (IV) fluids and will not be able to eat, as the colon needs time to recover. A colectomy rarely causes any major problems with digestive functions, and you should be able to eat after a few days (starting with clear liquids).

Sometimes the tumor is large and blocks the colon; in such cases, a colonoscope is used to put a stent (a hollow metal or plastic tube) inside the colon to relieve the blockage and help prepare for surgery a few days later.

If a stent cannot be placed or if the tumor has caused a hole in the colon, a temporary **colostomy** may be needed. This involves the same type of surgery as above, but instead of reconnecting the segments of the colon, the end of the colon is attached to an opening (**stoma**) in the abdomen for the purpose of getting rid of body wastes. A removable collecting bag is then connected to the stoma to hold the waste. Once you are healthier, another operation (known as a colostomy reversal) can be done to reattach the ends of the colon. Rarely, if a tumor cannot be removed or a stent placed, a permanent colostomy may be needed. For more information on colostomies, visit our Web site at **www.cancer.org**, or call **800-ACS-2345** and request the document *Colostomy: A Guide*.

Laparoscopic-assisted colectomy

This is a newer approach to removing part of the colon and nearby lymph nodes that may be an option for some earlier-stage cancers. Instead of making one long incision in the abdomen, the surgeon makes several smaller incisions. Special long instruments are inserted through these incisions to remove part of the colon and lymph nodes. One of the instruments has a small video camera on the end, which allows the surgeon to see inside the abdomen. Once the diseased part of the colon has been freed, one of the incisions is made larger to allow for its removal.

Because the incisions are smaller with laparoscopic-assisted colectomy than with a standard colectomy, they usually heal faster. Patients may recover slightly faster and have less pain than they do after standard colon surgery.

Laparoscopic-assisted surgery appears to be about as likely to be curative as the standard approach for earlier-stage cancer, but the surgery requires special expertise. If you are considering this approach, be sure to look for a skilled surgeon who has done a lot of these operations.

Polypectomy and local excision

Some early colon cancer (stage 0 and some early stage I tumors) or polyps can be removed by surgery through a colonoscope. When this is done, the surgeon does not have to cut into the abdomen. For a **polypectomy,** the cancer is cut out across the base of the polyp's stalk, the area that resembles the stem of a mushroom. **Local excision** removes superficial tumors and a small amount of nearby tissue.

Rectal Surgery

Surgery is usually the main treatment for rectal cancer, although radiation and chemotherapy will often be given before or after surgery. Several surgical methods are used for removing or destroying rectal cancer.

Polypectomy and local excision

These procedures, described on page 90 in the colon surgery section, can be used to remove superficial cancer or polyps. Both procedures are done with instruments inserted through the anus, without making a surgical opening in the skin of the abdomen.

Local transanal resection (full thickness resection)

As with polypectomy and local excision, local transanal resection is done with instruments inserted through the anus, without making an opening in the skin of the abdomen. This operation involves cutting through all layers of the rectum to remove invasive cancer, as well as some surrounding normal rectal tissue. This procedure can be used to remove some stage I rectal cancer in which the tumor is relatively small and not too far from the anus.

Low anterior resection

Some stage I rectal cancer and most stage II or III cancers in the upper two-thirds of the rectum (close to where it connects with the colon) can be removed by low anterior resection. In this procedure the tumor is removed without affecting the anus. After low anterior resection, your colon will be attached to the anus and your waste will leave the body in the usual way.

A low anterior resection is like most abdominal operations. You will need to take laxatives and enemas before surgery to empty the intestines. Just before surgery, you will be given general anesthesia, which puts you into a deep sleep. The surgeon makes the incision only in the abdomen. Then the surgeon removes the cancer and a margin of normal tissue on either side of the cancer, along with nearby lymph nodes and a large amount of fatty and fibrous tissue around the rectum. The colon is then reattached to the rectum that is remaining so that a colostomy is not necessary.

Sometimes, the entire rectum may be removed and the colon attached to the anus. This is called a coloanal anastomosis. This is a more difficult procedure, but modern techniques have made it possible. Sometimes when a coloanal anastomosis is done, a small pouch is made by doubling back a short segment of colon (called a colonic J-pouch) or by enlarging a segment (called coloplasty). This small reservoir of colon then functions like the rectum did before surgery. You may need to have a temporary colostomy opening for about 8 weeks while the bowel heals. A second operation is then done to close the colostomy opening.

Abdominoperineal resection

An **abdominoperineal (AP) resection** is more involved than a low anterior resection. It can be used to treat some stage I cancers and most stage II or III rectal cancers in the lower third of the rectum (the part nearest to the anus), especially if the cancer is growing into the **sphincter** (the muscle that keeps the anus closed and prevents stool leakage). Here, the surgeon makes one incision in the abdomen and another in the perineal area around the anus. This incision allows the surgeon to remove the anus and the tissues surrounding it, including the sphincter muscle. Because the anus is removed, you will need a permanent colostomy to allow stool a path out of the body.

The usual hospital stay for a low anterior resection or an AP resection is 4 to 7 days, depending on your overall health. Recovery time at home may be 3 to 6 weeks. If you have had a colostomy, you will need help in learning how to manage it. A specially trained ostomy nurse or **enterostomal therapist** can do this. This person will usually see you in the hospital before your operation to mark a site for the colostomy opening and later can come to your house or an outpatient setting to provide you with more training.

Pelvic exenteration

If the rectal cancer is growing into nearby organs, a **pelvic exenteration** may be recommended. This is an extensive operation. Not only will the surgeon remove the rectum, but also nearby organs such as the bladder, prostate (in men), or uterus (in women) if the cancer has spread to these organs. You will need a colostomy after pelvic exenteration. If the bladder is removed, you will also need a **urostomy** (an opening where urine exits the front of the abdomen and is held in a portable pouch).

Side Effects of Colorectal Surgery

Potential side effects of surgery depend on several factors, including the extent of the operation and a person's general health before surgery. Most people will have at least some pain after the operation, although this can usually be controlled with medicines if needed. Eating problems usually resolve within a few days after surgery.

Other problems may include bleeding from the surgery, blood clots in the legs, and damage to nearby organs during the operation. Rarely, the connections between the ends of the intestine may not hold together completely and may leak, which can lead to infection. It is also possible that the incision might open up. After the surgery, you might develop scar tissue that causes tissues in the abdomen to stick together. These are called **adhesions** and can sometimes cause pain. In rare cases, the adhesions can cause the bowel to become blocked, requiring further surgery.

Some people may require a temporary or permanent colostomy after surgery. This may take some time to get used to and may require some lifestyle adjustments. Your surgical team can help you learn what to expect.

Sexual impact of colorectal surgery

If you are a man, an AP resection may stop your erections or ability to reach orgasm. In other cases, your pleasure at orgasm may become less intense. Normal aging may cause some of these changes, but they may be made worse by the surgery.

An AP resection can also damage the nerves that control ejaculation, which can cause you to have little or no semen at orgasm (called dry ejaculation or dry orgasm). Sometimes the surgery causes retrograde ejaculation, which means the semen goes backward into the bladder. This distinction is important if you want to father a child, but otherwise, both conditions are relatively harmless. Retrograde ejaculation is less serious in regard to fertility because infertility specialists can recover sperm cells from the urine, which can then be used to fertilize an egg. If sperm cells cannot be recovered from your semen or urine, specialists may be able to retrieve them directly from the testicles by minor surgery and then use them for in vitro fertilization.

If you are a woman, most colorectal surgeries should not cause any loss of sexual function. Abdominal adhesions (scar tissue) may sometimes cause pain or discomfort during intercourse. Of course, if the uterus is removed, pregnancy will not be possible.

No matter your gender, a colostomy can have an impact on your body image and your sexual comfort level. While it may require some adjustments, it should not prevent you from having an enjoyable sex life.

For more information on dealing with the sexual impact of cancer and its treatment, call the American Cancer Society at **800-ACS-2345** and request *Sexuality and Cancer: For the Man Who Has Cancer and His Partner* or *Sexuality and Cancer: For the Woman Who Has Cancer and Her Partner.*

Surgical Treatment of Colorectal Cancer Metastases

Sometimes, surgery for cancer that has metasta-sized to other organs can help you live longer or, depending on the extent of the disease, may even cure you. If a small number of metastases have spread to only the liver or lungs (the most com-mon sites of metastases), they can sometimes be removed by surgery. This will depend on the size, number, and location of metastases.

In cases where surgical removal of tumors is not possible, nonsurgical treatments may be used to destroy (ablate) the tumors. These methods are less likely to be curative. Several different techniques may be used.

Radiofrequency ablation

In **radiofrequency ablation (RFA)**, a thin, needle-like probe placed through the skin and into the tumor releases high-energy radio waves into the tumor. Placement of the probe is guided by ultrasound or CT scans. The high-frequency current heats the tumor and destroys the cancer cells.

Ethanol (alcohol) ablation

Ethanol (alcohol) ablation, also known as **percutaneous ethanol injection (PEI),** involves injecting concentrated alcohol directly into the tumor to kill cancer cells. The alcohol is usually injected through the skin by using a needle, which is guided by ultrasound or computed tomography.

Cryosurgery

Cryosurgery destroys a tumor by freezing it with a very cold metal probe. The probe is guided into the tumor by using ultrasound. This method can be used to treat larger tumors than either of the other ablation techniques described above, but sometimes requires general anesthesia.

Since these 3 treatments usually do not require surgery to remove any part of the liver, they are often good options for patients whose disease is not curable with surgery.

Hepatic artery embolization

Another option for tumors in the liver that cannot be removed, **hepatic artery embolization** reduces the blood flow in the hepatic artery, the artery through which most cancer cells feed into the liver. The doctor injects materials that block the artery. As a result, the tumor does not get as much blood, reducing its growth. Most healthy liver cells will not be affected, as most get their blood supply from the portal vein, not the hepatic artery.

Hepatic artery embolization involves putting a catheter into an artery in the inner thigh and threading it up into the liver. A dye is usually injected into the bloodstream to allow the doctor to monitor the path of the catheter via angiography, a special type of imaging procedure. Once the catheter is in place, small particles are injected into the artery to block it.

Embolization also reduces some of the blood supply to the normal liver tissue. This may be dangerous for patients with diseases such as hepatitis and cirrhosis that are affecting the part of the liver not affected by cancer.

Radiation Therapy

Radiation therapy uses high-energy rays (such as x-rays) or particles to destroy cancer cells. It may be used as part of treatment for either colon or rectal cancer. Chemotherapy (see pages 101–103) can make radiation therapy more effective against some colon and rectal cancers, and these 2 treatments are often used together.

In people with colon cancer, radiation therapy is mainly used when the cancer has attached to an internal organ or the lining of the abdomen. In those circumstances, the surgeon may not be able to be certain that all the cancer has been removed, and radiation therapy may be used to kill any cancer cells remaining after surgery. Radiation therapy is seldom used to treat metastatic colon cancer because of its side effects, which limit the dose that can be used.

For rectal cancer, radiation therapy is usually given to help prevent the cancer from coming back in the pelvis. It may be given either before or after surgery, but recently doctors have begun to favor preoperative treatment, along with chemotherapy. If the size of the rectal cancer or the position of it makes surgery difficult, use of radiation may shrink the tumor, making surgery more likely to be successful.

Radiation therapy can also be given to help control rectal cancer in people who are not healthy enough for surgery. In addition, radiation may be used to ease symptoms in people with advanced cancer that is causing intestinal blockage, bleeding, or pain.

Types of Radiation Therapy
Different types of radiation therapy can be used to treat colon and rectal cancers.

External-beam radiation therapy (for colon cancer)
External beam radiation therapy focuses radiation on the cancer from a machine called a **linear accelerator,** which is outside the body. This is the type of radiation therapy most often recommended for people with colon cancer.

Before treatments start, the radiation team takes careful measurements to determine the correct angles for aiming the radiation beams and the proper dose of radiation. External radiation therapy is much like getting an x-ray, but the radiation is more intense. The procedure itself is painless. Each treatment lasts only a few minutes, although the setup time—getting the patient positioned for treatment—usually takes longer. Radiation treatments are usually given 5 days a week for several weeks.

Endocavitary radiation therapy (for rectal cancer)
As with external-beam radiation therapy, this therapy is delivered from a radiation source outside the body. A hand-held device is placed into the anus and delivers high-intensity radiation

over a few minutes. This is repeated about 3 more times at about 2-week intervals. The advantage of this approach is that the radiation reaches the rectum without passing through the skin and other abdominal tissues, which means it is less likely to cause side effects. This can allow some patients, particularly elderly persons, to avoid radical surgery and colostomy. It is used only for small tumors. Sometimes external-beam radiation therapy is also given.

Brachytherapy

Brachytherapy is a type of **internal radiation therapy** that uses small pellets of radioactive material placed next to or directly into the cancer. The radiation travels only a short distance, limiting the effects on surrounding healthy tissues. Internal radiation is sometimes used in treating people with rectal cancer, particularly people who are not healthy enough to tolerate curative surgery. This is generally a one-time only procedure and does not require daily visits for several weeks.

Side Effects of Radiation Therapy

If you will be undergoing radiation therapy, speak with your doctor beforehand about possible side effects so you will know what to expect. These are some of the potential side effects of radiation therapy for colon and rectal cancer:

- mild skin irritation at the site where radiation beams were aimed
- nausea

- rectal irritation, which can cause diarrhea, painful bowel movements, or blood in the stool
- bowel incontinence
- bladder irritation, which can cause frequent urination, incontinence, burning sensations while urinating, or blood in the urine
- fatigue
- sexual problems (impotence in men and vaginal irritation in women)

Most side effects should lessen after treatments are completed, but problems such as rectal and bladder irritation and sexual side effects may persist. Some degree of rectal and/or bladder irritation may be a permanent side effect. If these or other side effects begin to develop, talk to your doctor right away so steps can be taken to reduce or relieve them.

Chemotherapy

Chemotherapy, or chemo, is treatment with anti-cancer drugs. Systemic chemotherapy uses drugs that are injected into a vein or given by mouth. These drugs enter the bloodstream and reach all areas of the body. This treatment is useful for cancer that has spread beyond the organ in which it started. In regional chemotherapy, drugs are injected directly into an artery leading to a part of the body containing a tumor. This approach of using a concentrated dose of chemotherapy to target the cancer cells reduces side effects by limiting the amount reaching the rest of the body. **Hepatic arterial infusion,** in which chemotherapy is given directly into the hepatic artery, is an example of regional chemotherapy sometimes used for colon cancer that has spread to the liver.

There are several situations in which chemotherapy may be used to treat colon or rectal cancer.

Chemotherapy after surgery

The use of chemotherapy after surgery, known as **adjuvant chemotherapy,** can increase the survival rate for patients with some stages of colon cancer and rectal cancer. Adjuvant chemotherapy is given when there is no evidence of cancer remaining but there is a chance that the cancer might come back. The theory behind adjuvant therapy is that a small number of cancer cells may not have been removed by surgery or may have broken away from the primary tumor and settled in other parts of the body. The hope is that the chemotherapy can kill these cells, wherever they may be.

Chemotherapy before surgery

For some patients with rectal cancer, chemotherapy is given (along with radiation) before surgery to try to shrink the cancer and make surgery easier. This is known as **neoadjuvant chemotherapy.**

Chemotherapy for advanced cancer

Chemotherapy can also be used to help shrink tumors and relieve symptoms for patients with more advanced cancer. Although it is very unlikely to be curative in such situations, it may greatly extend survival time for some patients.

Drugs Used to Treat Colorectal Cancer

Several drugs can be used to treat colorectal cancer. Often, 2 or more of these drugs are combined to be more effective.

5-FU (fluorouracil)

Fluorouracil or 5-FU has been used for several decades and is part of most chemotherapy regimens for colorectal cancer. It is often given with another drug called leucovorin (also called folinic acid), which increases its effectiveness.

Your doctor may prescribe 5-FU according to one of several dosing schedules. It can be given as an intravenous (IV) infusion over 2 hours, or (more commonly) as a quick injection followed by continuous IV infusion over 1 or 2 days. For continuous infusions, the patient wears a small, battery-operated pump that infuses 5-FU into an IV catheter. For most chemotherapy regimens, treatment with 5-FU is repeated every 2 weeks, over a period of 6 months to a year.

The possible side effects of this drug include nausea, loss of appetite, mouth sores, diarrhea, low blood cell counts, sensitivity to sunlight, and a syndrome of hand and foot redness that is sometimes accompanied by blistering or skin peeling.

Capecitabine (Xeloda)

Capecitabine (Xeloda) is a chemotherapy drug in pill form (rather than IV). It is usually taken twice a day for 2 weeks, followed by a week off.

Capecitabine changes to 5-FU when it gets to the tumor site. The effectiveness of this drug is similar to that of giving 5-FU by continuous IV infusion.

Whereas this drug may be taken at home as a pill, it is still a strong chemotherapy medicine. The possible side effects are similar to those listed for regular 5-FU. Although most of the side effects appear to be less common with this drug than with regular 5-FU, the hand and foot problems described on page 103 are more common.

Irinotecan (Camptosar)

Irinotecan is often combined with 5-FU and leucovorin (known as the FOLFIRI regimen) as a **first-line treatment** for advanced colorectal cancer. In some cases, it may be tried by itself as a **second-line treatment** if other chemotherapy drugs are no longer effective. It is given as an IV infusion for 30 minutes to 2 hours.

One problem with irinotecan is that some people who have a certain inherited genetic variation are unable to metabolize (break down) the drug, so it stays in the body and causes severe side effects. The simplest way to test for the genetic variation is to measure the blood level of bilirubin, a substance made in the liver. If bilirubin is slightly elevated, this can be a sign of the variation that makes people sensitive to irinotecan. So far, most doctors are not routinely testing for the genetic variant itself.

The major possible side effects of irinotecan are severe diarrhea and low blood counts, although other effects such as nausea are possible as well.

Your doctor will likely give you medicine to take before treatment to help prevent diarrhea. You need to tell your doctor right away if you develop diarrhea or any other side effects. Your doctor may not advise irinotecan if you are elderly or have serious health problems. In rare cases, severe side effects can even be fatal.

Oxaliplatin (Eloxatin)

This drug is usually combined with 5-FU and leucovorin (known as the FOLFOX regimen) or with capecitabine (known as the CapeOX regimen) as a first- or second-line treatment for advanced colorectal cancer. It may also be used as adjuvant therapy after surgery for earlier stage cancer. Oxaliplatin is given as an IV infusion over 2 hours, usually once every 2 or 3 weeks.

Oxaliplatin can affect peripheral nerves, which can cause numbness, tingling, and intense sensitivity to temperature in the extremities, especially the hands and feet. In most patients, this side effect goes away after treatment has stopped, but in some cases it can cause long-lasting nerve damage. If oxaliplatin is prescribed for you, talk with your doctor about side effects beforehand, and let him or her know as soon as you develop numbness and tingling or other side effects.

Side Effects of Chemotherapy

Chemotherapy drugs work by attacking cells that are dividing quickly, which is why they work against cancer cells. But other cells in the body, such as those in the bone marrow, the lining of the mouth and intestines, and the hair follicles, also divide quickly. These cells are also likely to be affected by chemotherapy and lead to side effects.

The side effects of chemotherapy depend on the type and dose of drugs given and the length of time they are taken. These are some of the general side effects of chemotherapy:

- hair loss
- mouth sores
- loss of appetite
- nausea and vomiting
- increased chance of infections (because of low white blood cell counts)
- easy bruising or bleeding (because of low blood platelet counts)
- fatigue (because of low red blood cell counts)

Along with these possible reactions, some side effects are specific to certain medicines. These are discussed above in the descriptions of the individual drugs.

Most side effects are short-term and tend to go away after treatment is finished. There are often ways to lessen side effects. For example, drugs can be given to help prevent or reduce nausea and vomiting. Do not hesitate to discuss any questions about side effects with your cancer care team.

If you experience any side effects or notice changes while receiving chemotherapy, report these to your medical team right away so that they can be treated promptly. In some cases, the doses of the chemotherapy drugs may need to be reduced or treatment may need to be delayed or stopped to prevent side effects from getting worse.

Elderly people seem to be able to tolerate chemotherapy for colorectal cancer fairly well. There is no reason to withhold treatment in otherwise healthy people simply because of age.

For more general information about chemotherapy, call the American Cancer Society at **800-ACS-2345** and request the document *Understanding Chemotherapy: A Guide for Patients and Families,* or visit our Web site, **www.cancer.org**.

Targeted Therapies

As researchers have learned more about the gene and protein changes in the body that cause cancer, they have been able to develop newer drugs that specifically target these changes. These targeted drugs work differently than standard chemotherapy drugs and often have different (and less severe) side effects. Currently, targeted therapies are most often used either with chemotherapy or alone if chemotherapy is no longer working.

Bevacizumab (Avastin)

Bevacizumab is a manmade version of an immune system protein called a **monoclonal antibody.** This antibody targets (works against) **vascular endothelial growth factor (VEGF),** a protein that helps tumors form new blood vessels to get nutrients (a process known as **angiogenesis**).

By reducing the formation of new blood vessels to the tumor, bevacizumab can limit the growth of the tumor. Bevacizumab is most often used along with chemotherapy drugs as a first- or second-line treatment for metastatic colorectal cancer.

Bevacizumab is given by intravenous (IV) infusion, usually once every 2 or 3 weeks. While it has been shown to help improve survival when added to chemotherapy, it can also add to side effects. Rare, but possibly serious side effects include blood clots, holes forming in the colon (requiring surgery to correct), heart problems, and slow wound healing. More common side effects include high blood pressure, tiredness, bleeding, low white blood cell counts, headaches, mouth sores, loss of appetite, and diarrhea.

Cetuximab (Erbitux)

Cetuximab is a monoclonal antibody that specifically attacks the **epidermal growth factor receptor (EGFR)**, a molecule that often appears in high amounts on the surface of cancer cells and helps them grow. By attacking EGFR, cetuximab can limit the growth of cancer cells.

Cetuximab is used in metastatic colorectal cancer, usually after other treatments have been tried and are no longer successful. It can be used either with irinotecan or by itself in those who cannot take irinotecan or whose cancer is no longer responding to it.

Cetuximab is given by IV infusion, usually once a week. A rare, but serious side effect of cetuximab is an allergic reaction during the first infusion, which could cause low blood pressure and problems with breathing. You may be given medicine before treatment to help prevent this. Other, less serious side effects may include an acne-like rash, headache, tiredness, fever, and diarrhea.

Panitumumab (Vectibix)

Panitumumab is another monoclonal antibody that attacks colorectal cancer cells. Like cetuximab, it targets the EGFR protein. It is used alone to treat metastatic colorectal cancer after other treatments have been tried and are no longer working.

Panitumumab is given by IV infusion, usually once every 2 weeks. Most people develop skin problems such as a rash during treatment, which in some cases can lead to an infection. Other possible serious side effects are lung scarring and allergic reactions. Sensitivity to sunlight, fatigue, diarrhea, and changes in fingernails and toenails are also possible.

Treatment by Stage of Colon Cancer

For colon cancer that has not spread to distant sites, surgery is usually the primary or first treatment. Adjuvant chemotherapy may also be used. Most adjuvant treatment is given for about 6 months.

Treatment for Stage 0 Colon Cancer

Since stage 0 cancer has not grown beyond the inner lining of the colon, surgery to take out the cancer is all that is needed. This may be done in many cases by polypectomy or local excision through a colonoscope. Colon resection may be needed if a tumor is too big to be removed by local excision.

Treatment for Stage I Colon Cancer

Stage I colon cancer has grown through several layers of the colon, but it has not spread beyond the colon wall itself. Colectomy—surgery to remove the section of colon containing cancer and nearby lymph nodes—is the standard treatment. You do not need any additional therapy.

Treatment for Stage II Colon Cancer

Stage II colon cancer has grown through the wall of the colon and may extend into nearby tissue. It has not yet spread to the lymph nodes.

Colectomy—surgery to remove the section of colon containing cancer and nearby lymph nodes—is usually the only treatment needed. If your doctor thinks your cancer is likely to come back because of how it looks under the microscope or other factors, adjuvant chemotherapy may be recommended. Chemotherapy is not standard treatment for this stage of colon cancer, but many doctors recommend it if the risk for recurrence seems high, such as in stage IIB disease. There are clinical trials studying whether chemotherapy should be recommended for stage IIB disease (and if so, what regimen), and you might consider enrolling in one. Doctors aren't sure which chemotherapy regimen might be best in this situation. Some of the more commonly used treatments include FOLFOX

(5-FU, leucovorin, and oxaliplatin), 5-FU and leucovorin alone, or capecitabine. Your doctor may recommend one of these treatment regimens if it is better suited to your health needs.

If your surgeon is not sure he or she was able to remove all of the cancer because it was growing into other tissues, radiation therapy may be recommended to kill any remaining cancer cells. Radiation therapy can be given to the area of your abdomen where the cancer was growing.

Treatment for Stage III Colon Cancer

Stage III colon cancer has spread to nearby lymph nodes, but it has not yet spread to other parts of the body.

Colectomy—surgery to remove the section of colon containing cancer and nearby lymph nodes—followed by adjuvant chemotherapy is the standard treatment. The FOLFOX regimen is the most common chemotherapy combination, although some doctors may prefer 5-FU and leucovorin, capecitabine and oxaliplatin (CapeOX), or capecitabine alone if they are better suited to your health needs.

Your doctors may also recommend radiation therapy if your surgeon believes cancer may still be present after surgery.

Treatment for Stage IV Colon Cancer

Stage IV colon cancer has spread from the colon to distant organs and tissues such as the liver, lungs, peritoneum, or ovaries.

Surgery in stage IV colon cancer is usually not done with the expectation of curing the disease. However, if only a few small metastases (usually 5 or fewer) are present in the liver or lung and can be completely removed along with the colon cancer, surgery can help you live longer and may even cure you. In such circumstances, surgery is usually followed by chemotherapy. In some cases, hepatic arterial infusion may be used if the tumors were in the liver. If the metastases cannot be surgically removed because they are too large or there are too many of them, chemotherapy may be tried first to shrink the tumors to a size at which surgical removal is possible. Chemotherapy would be given again after surgery. Another option may be to destroy tumors in the liver with cryosurgery, radiofrequency ablation, or other nonsurgical methods.

If the cancer is too widespread to be cured or treated solely with surgery, operations such as a segmental resection or diverting colostomy might still be used in some cases to relieve or prevent blockage of the colon and to prevent other local complications. In some patients with extensive spread of cancer, such a blockage can be prevented or managed by inserting a stent (a hollow metal or plastic tube) into the colon during colonoscopy to keep it open so that surgery can be avoided.

Most patients with stage IV cancer will get chemotherapy and/or targeted therapies to control the cancer. The most commonly used regimens include the following:

- FOLFOX (5-FU, leucovorin, and oxaliplatin), with or without bevacizumab
- FOLFIRI (5-FU, leucovorin, and irinotecan), with or without bevacizumab
- CapeOX (capecitabine and oxaliplatin), with or without bevacizumab
- 5-FU and leucovorin, with or without bevacizumab
- capecitabine, with or without bevacizumab
- irinotecan, with or without cetuximab
- cetuximab alone
- panitumumab alone

The choice of regimens may depend on several factors, including any previous treatments you have had and your overall health. If one of these regimens is no longer effective, another may be tried.

Treatment for Recurrent Colon Cancer

Recurrent cancer means that the cancer has returned after treatment. The **recurrence** may be local (near the area of the initial tumor), or it may affect distant organs.

If the cancer comes back locally, surgery (followed by chemotherapy) can sometimes help you live longer and may even cure you. If the cancer cannot be removed surgically, chemotherapy may be tried first. If it shrinks the tumor enough, surgery may be an option at this point. Surgery would again be followed by more chemotherapy.

If the cancer comes back in a distant site, it is most likely to appear first in the liver. Surgery may be an option in some cases. If not, chemotherapy may be tried first to shrink the tumor(s), followed by surgery. If the cancer is too widespread to be treated surgically, chemotherapy and/or targeted therapies may be used. Possible regimens are the same as for stage IV disease. The options depend on which drugs you received before the cancer came back and how long ago you received them, as well as your overall health. Surgery may still be needed at some point to relieve or prevent blockage of the colon and to prevent other local complications.

Because recurrent cancer can often be difficult to treat, you may also want to speak with your doctor about clinical trials for which you might be eligible.

Treatment by Stage of Rectal Cancer

For rectal cancer that has not spread to distant sites, surgery is usually the primary or first treatment. Adjuvant treatment with radiation and chemotherapy may also be used. Most adjuvant treatment is given for about 6 months.

Treatment for Stage 0 Rectal Cancer

Stage 0 rectal cancer has not grown beyond the inner lining of the rectum. Removing or destroying the cancer is all that is needed. You can be treated with a polypectomy, local excision, or transanal resection. You will need no further treatment.

If you are too sick to withstand surgery, you may be treated only with radiation therapy such as endocavitary radiation therapy (aiming radiation through the anus) or brachytherapy (placing radioactive pellets directly into the cancer), although it is not clear if this is as effective as surgery.

Treatment for Stage I Rectal Cancer

In stage I rectal cancer, the cancer has grown through the first layer of the rectum into deeper layers but has not spread beyond the rectal wall itself.

Surgery is the main treatment at this stage. Either a low anterior resection or an abdomino-perineal resection may be done, depending on exactly where the cancer is found within the rectum. Adjuvant therapy is not needed after these operations, unless the surgeon finds the cancer is more advanced than was thought before surgery.

For some small stage I rectal cancers, another option may be removing them through the anus (transanal resection), without an abdominal incision. In most cases, adjuvant therapy with radiation and chemotherapy (usually 5-FU) is advised for patients having such surgery.

If you are too sick to withstand surgery, you may be treated with only radiation therapy, such as endocavitary radiation therapy (aiming radiation through the anus) or brachytherapy (placing radioactive pellets directly into the cancer). However, this has not been proven to be as effective as surgery.

Treatment for Stage II Rectal Cancer

At stage II rectal cancer, the cancer has grown through the wall of the rectum and into nearby tissues. It has not yet spread to the lymph nodes.

Stage II rectal cancer is usually treated by low anterior resection or abdominoperineal resection (depending on where the cancer is in the rectum), along with both chemotherapy and radiation therapy. Radiation can be given either before or after surgery. Many doctors now favor giving radiation therapy and chemotherapy before surgery (called neoadjuvant treatment), as well as giving adjuvant chemotherapy after surgery. Common chemotherapy regimens include the FOLFOX regimen (5-FU, leucovorin, and oxaliplatin), 5-FU and leucovorin, capecitabine and oxaliplatin (CapeOX), or capecitabine alone, based on what is best suited to your health needs.

If neoadjuvant therapy shrinks the tumor enough, in some cases a transanal resection can be done instead of a more invasive low anterior resection or abdominoperineal resection. This may avert the need for a colostomy. A problem with this less invasive surgery is there is no way to know whether the cancer has spread further into the pelvis or to lymph nodes. For this reason, a transanal resection is not generally recommended.

Treatment for Stage III Rectal Cancer

In stage III, the cancer has spread to nearby lymph nodes but not to other parts of the body.

The rectal tumor is usually removed by low anterior resection or abdominoperineal resection. In rare cases where the cancer has reached nearby organs, a pelvic exenteration may be needed. Radiation therapy is given before or after surgery. As in stage II, many doctors now prefer to give radiation therapy and chemotherapy before surgery because it lowers the chance that the cancer will come back in the pelvis. For larger tumors, neoadjuvant chemotherapy and radiation may also make the surgery more effective.

At this stage, chemotherapy is also given after surgery. The most common regimens include FOLFOX (oxaliplatin, 5-FU, and leucovorin), 5-FU and leucovorin, capecitabine and oxaliplatin (CapeOX), or capecitabine alone. Your doctor may recommend one treatment regimen in particular if it is better suited to your health needs.

Treatment for Stage IV Rectal Cancer

In stage IV rectal cancer, the cancer has spread to distant organs and tissues such as the liver or lungs. Treatment options for stage IV disease depend to some extent on how widespread the cancer is.

If there is a chance that all of the cancer can be removed (for example, there are only a few tumors in the liver or lungs), there are several treatment options:

- surgery to remove the rectal lesion and distant tumors, followed by chemotherapy (and radiation therapy in some cases)
- chemotherapy, followed by surgery to remove the rectal lesion and distant tumors, usually followed by more chemotherapy and radiation therapy
- chemotherapy and radiation therapy, followed by surgery to remove the rectal lesion and distant tumors, followed by chemotherapy

Treatment may help you live longer and in some cases may even cure you. Surgery to remove the rectal tumor would usually be a low anterior resection or abdominoperineal (AP) resection, depending on where it is located. If you have only liver metastases, you may be treated with chemotherapy given directly into the hepatic artery (called hepatic arterial infusion). This treatment method shrinks the cancer in the liver more effectively than chemotherapy given intravenously.

If the cancer is too widespread to be completely removed by surgery, treatment options may depend on whether the cancer is causing any symptoms. Widespread cancer that is not causing symptoms is usually treated with chemotherapy. These are the most commonly used regimens:

- FOLFOX (5-FU, leucovorin, and oxaliplatin), with or without bevacizumab
- FOLFIRI (5-FU, leucovorin, and irinotecan), with or without bevacizumab
- CapeOX (capecitabine and oxaliplatin), with or without bevacizumab
- 5-FU and leucovorin, with or without bevacizumab
- capecitabine, with or without bevacizumab
- irinotecan, with or without cetuximab
- cetuximab alone
- panitumumab alone

The choice of regimens may depend on several factors, including any previous treatments and your overall health and ability to tolerate treatment.

If the chemotherapy shrinks the tumors, it may be possible to consider surgery to try to remove all of the cancer at this point. Cancer that does not shrink with chemotherapy and widespread cancer that is causing symptoms are unlikely to be cured, and treatment is aimed at relieving symptoms and avoiding long-term complications such as bleeding or blockage of the intestines. These are some of the possible treatments:

- surgical resection of the rectal tumor
- surgery to create a colostomy and bypass the rectal tumor
- use of a special laser to destroy the tumor within the rectum
- placement of a stent (a hollow plastic or metal tube) within the rectum to keep it open; this does not require surgery
- radiation therapy and chemotherapy
- chemotherapy alone

If tumors in the liver cannot be removed by surgery because they are too large or there are too many of them, it may be possible to destroy them by freezing (cryosurgery), heating (radiofrequency ablation), or vaporizing the tumor with a laser (**photocoagulation**), or with other nonsurgical methods.

Treatment for Recurrent Rectal Cancer

Recurrent cancer means that the cancer has returned after treatment. It may come back locally (near the area of the initial rectal tumor) or in distant organs. Most recurrences develop in the first 2 to 3 years after surgery. If the cancer comes back locally, chemotherapy and radiation therapy aimed at the tumor may be given if radiation therapy was not used before. Surgery to remove the cancer is used if possible. In some cases surgery may be followed by radiation therapy.

If the cancer comes back in a distant site, treatment depends on whether it can be removed by surgery. If the cancer can be removed, surgery is done to remove the tumor. This is followed by chemotherapy (see "Treatment for Stage IV Rectal Cancer" on page 117 for a list of possible regimens). If the patient has not received chemotherapy within the last year, neoadjuvant chemotherapy can be given before surgery as well. If cancer has spread to the liver, chemotherapy may be given into the hepatic artery (called hepatic arterial infusion). This treatment method shrinks the cancer in the liver more effectively than chemotherapy given intravenously.

If the cancer has recurred in a distant site and cannot be removed by surgery, chemotherapy is usually the first option. The regimen used will depend on what the patient has received previously and on his or her overall health. If the cancer shrinks, surgery may be an option in some cases. This would be followed by more chemotherapy.

As with stage IV cancer, surgery or other approaches may be used at some point to relieve symptoms and avoid long-term complications such as bleeding or blockage of the intestines.

As recurrent cancer can often be difficult to treat, you may also want to speak with your doctor about clinical trials for which you might be eligible.

Clinical Trials

If you've been told you have cancer, you have probably already had a lot of decisions to make. One of the most important decisions you will make is deciding which treatment is best for you. You may have heard about **clinical trials** being done for your type of cancer. Or maybe someone on your cancer care team has mentioned a clinical trial to you. Clinical trials can be one way to get state-of-the art cancer care, but they are not right for everyone.

Here, we will give you a brief review of clinical trials. Talking to your cancer care team, your family, and your friends can help you make the best treatment choice for you.

What Are Clinical Trials?

Clinical trials are carefully controlled research studies that are done with patients. These studies test whether a new treatment is safe and how well it works in patients; additionally, the studies may test new ways to diagnose or prevent a disease. Clinical trials have led to many advances in cancer prevention, diagnosis, and treatment.

Clinical trials are done to get a closer look at promising new treatments or procedures in patients. A clinical trial is only done when there is good reason to believe that the treatment, test, or procedure being studied may be better than the one used now. Treatments used in clinical trials are often found to have real benefits and may go on to become tomorrow's **standard therapy.**

Clinical trials can focus on many things:

- new uses of drugs that are already approved by the **U.S. Food and Drug Administration (FDA)**
- new drugs that have not yet been approved by the FDA
- nondrug treatments (such as radiation therapy)
- medical procedures (such as types of surgery)
- herbs and vitamins
- tools to improve the ways medicines or diagnostic tests are used
- medicines or procedures to relieve symptoms or improve comfort
- combinations of treatments and procedures

Researchers conduct studies of new treatments to try to answer the following questions:

- Is the treatment helpful?
- What is the best way to give it?
- Does it work better than other treatments already available?
- What side effects does the treatment cause?
- Are there more or fewer side effects than the standard treatment used now?
- Do the benefits outweigh the side effects?
- In which patients is the treatment most likely to be helpful?

Phases of Clinical Trials

There are 4 phases of clinical trials, which are numbered I, II, III, and IV. We will use the example of testing a new cancer treatment drug to look at what each phase is like.

Phase I clinical trials

The purpose of a phase I study is to find the best way to give a new treatment safely to patients. The cancer care team closely watches patients for any harmful side effects.

For phase I studies, the drug has already been tested in laboratory and animal studies, but the side effects in patients are not fully known. Doctors start by giving very low doses of the drug to the first patients and increase the doses for later groups of patients until side effects appear or the desired effect is seen. Doctors are hoping to help patients, but the main purpose of a phase I trial is to test the safety of the drug.

Phase I clinical trials are often done in small groups of people with different types of cancer that have not responded to standard treatment or that keep coming back (recurring) after treatment. If a drug is found to be reasonably safe in phase I studies, it can be tested in a phase II clinical trial.

Phase II clinical trials

These studies are designed to learn whether the drug works. Patients are given the best dose as determined from phase I studies. They are closely watched for an effect on the cancer. The cancer care team also looks for side effects.

Phase II trials are often done in larger groups of patients with a specific cancer type that has not responded to standard treatment. If a drug is found to be effective in phase II studies, it can be tested in a phase III clinical trial.

Phase III clinical trials

Phase III studies involve large numbers of patients—most often those who have just been diagnosed with a specific type of cancer. Phase III clinical trials may enroll thousands of patients.

Often, these studies are **randomized.** This means that patients are randomly put in 1 of 2 (or more) groups. One group (called the **control group**) gets the standard, most accepted treatment. The other group(s) gets the new one(s) being studied. All patients in phase III studies are closely watched. The study will be stopped early if the side effects of the new treatment are too severe or if one group has much better results than the others.

Phase III clinical trials are usually needed before the FDA will approve a treatment for use by the general public.

Phase IV clinical trials

Once a drug has been approved by the FDA and is available for all patients, it is still studied in other clinical trials (sometimes referred to as phase IV studies). This way, more can be learned about short-term and long-term side effects and safety as the drug is used in larger numbers of patients with many types of diseases. Doctors can also learn more about how well the drug works and whether it might be helpful when used in other ways (such as in combination with other treatments).

Taking Part in a Clinical Trial

If you are in a clinical trial, you will have a team of experts taking care of you and watching your progress very carefully. Depending on the phase of the clinical trial, you may receive more attention (such as having more doctor visits and laboratory tests) than you would if you were treated outside of a clinical trial. Clinical trials are specially designed to pay close attention to you.

However, there are some risks. No one involved in the study knows in advance whether the treatment will work or exactly what side effects will occur. That is what the study is designed to find out. While most side effects go away in time, some may be long-lasting or even life-threatening. Keep in mind, though, that even standard treatments have side effects. Depending on many factors, you may decide to enter a clinical trial.

If you would like to take part in a clinical trial, you should begin by asking your doctor whether your clinic or hospital conducts clinical trials. There are requirements you must meet to take part in any clinical trial. The choice to enroll in a clinical trial is yours.

Your doctors and nurses will explain the study to you in detail. They will go over the possible risks and benefits and give you a form to read and sign. The form says that you understand the clinical trial and want to take part in it. This process is known as giving your **informed consent.** Even after reading and signing the form and after the clinical trial begins, you are free to leave the study at any time, for any reason. Taking part in a clinical trial does not keep you from getting other medical care you may need.

To find out more about clinical trials, talk to your cancer care team. Here are some questions you might ask:

- Is there a clinical trial for which I would be eligible?
- What is the purpose of the study?
- What kinds of tests and treatments does the study involve?
- What does this treatment do? Has it been used before?
- Will I know which treatment I receive?
- What is likely to happen in my case with, or without, this new treatment?
- What are my other choices and their pros and cons?
- How could the study affect my daily life?
- What side effects can I expect from the study? Can the side effects be controlled?
- Will I have to stay in the hospital? If so, how often and for how long?
- Will the study cost me anything? Will any of the treatment be free?
- If I am harmed as a result of the research, to what treatment would I be entitled?
- What type of long-term follow-up care is part of the study?
- Has the treatment been used to treat other types of cancer?

How Can I Find Out More About Clinical Trials That Might Be Right for Me?

The American Cancer Society offers a clinical trials matching service for patients and their family and friends. You can access this service on our Web site at **http://clinicaltrials.cancer.org** or by calling **800-303-5691**.

Based on the information you give about your cancer type, stage, and previous treatments, this service can put together a list of clinical trials that match your medical needs. The service will also ask where you live and whether you are willing to travel so that it can look for possible treatment centers.

You can also get a list of current clinical trials by calling the National Cancer Institute's (NCI's) Cancer Information Service at **800-4-CANCER** (**800-422-6237**) or by visiting the NCI clinical trials Web site at **www.cancer.gov/clinicaltrials**.

For more information, call the American Cancer Society at **800-ACS-2345** and request the document *Clinical Trials: What You Need to Know* or visit our Web site, **www.cancer.org**.

Complementary and Alternative Therapies

You have likely heard about ways to treat your cancer or relieve symptoms that are different from mainstream medical treatment. The wide variety of available methods include vitamins, herbs, special diets, acupuncture, and massage, among many others. You may have a lot of questions about these treatments. Here are some you may have thought of already:

- How do I know if a nonstandard treatment is safe?

- How do I know if it works?
- Should I try one or more of these treatments?
- What does my doctor know/think about these methods? Should I tell the doctor that I'm thinking about trying them?
- Will these treatments cause a problem with my standard medical treatment?
- What is the difference between "complementary" and "alternative" treatments?
- Where can I find out more about these treatments?

Not everyone uses the terms complementary and alternative the same way, so it can be confusing. The American Cancer Society uses the term **complementary therapy** to refer to medicines or methods that are used *along with* your regular medical care. An **alternative therapy** is a treatment used *instead of* standard medical treatment.

Complementary methods

Complementary treatment methods, for the most part, are not presented as cures for cancer. Most often they are used to help you feel better. Some methods that can be used in a complementary way are meditation to reduce stress, acupuncture to relieve pain, or peppermint tea to relieve nausea. There are many others. Some of these methods are known to help, while others have not been tested. Some have proved to have no helpful effects. A few have even been found harmful. However, some of these methods may add to your comfort and well-being.

You can safely use many complementary methods along with your medical treatment to help relieve symptoms or side effects, to ease pain, and to help you enjoy life more. For example, some people find methods such as aromatherapy, massage therapy, meditation, or yoga to be useful.

Alternative treatments

Alternative treatments are those that are used instead of standard medical care. These treatments have not been proved to be safe and effective in clinical trials. Some of these methods may be dangerous, and some have life-threatening side effects. The biggest danger in most cases is that you may lose the chance to benefit from standard treatment because of time spent pursuing alternative therapies. Delays or interruptions in your standard medical treatment may give the cancer more time to grow.

Considering Your Options

It is easy to see why someone with cancer would consider alternative methods. You want to do all you can to fight the cancer. Sometimes mainstream treatments such as chemotherapy can be hard to take, or they may no longer be working.

Sometimes people suggest that their method can cure your cancer without having serious side effects, and it is normal to want to believe them. The truth is that most nonstandard methods of treatment have not been tested and found to be effective for treating cancer.

As you consider your options, here are 3 important steps you can take:

- Talk to your doctor or nurse about any method you are thinking about using.
- Check the list of "red flags" below.
- Contact the American Cancer Society at **800-ACS-2345** to learn more about complementary and alternative methods in general and to learn more about the specific methods you are thinking about.

Red flags

Use the questions below to spot treatments or methods to avoid. A "yes" answer to any of these questions should raise a red flag:

- Does the treatment promise a cure for all or most types of cancer?
- Are you told not to use standard medical treatment?
- Is the treatment or drug a "secret" that only certain people can give?
- Does the treatment require you to travel to another country?
- Do the promoters attack the medical or scientific community?

The decision is yours

Decisions about how to treat or manage your cancer are always yours to make. If you are thinking about using a complementary or alternative therapy, be sure to learn about the method and talk with your doctor about it. With reliable information and the support of your cancer care team, you should be able to take advantage of the methods that can help you and avoid those that could be harmful.

More Treatment Information

For more details on treatment options, the National Comprehensive Cancer Network (NCCN) and the National Cancer Institute (NCI) are good sources of information.

The NCCN, made up of experts from the nation's leading cancer centers, develops cancer treatment guidelines for doctors to use when treating patients. Those are available on the NCCN Web site (**www.nccn.org**).

The American Cancer Society collaborates with the NCCN to produce a version of these treatment guidelines for colorectal cancer, written specifically for patients and their families. This less technical version is available on both the NCCN Web site (**www.nccn.org**) and the American Cancer Society Web site (**www.cancer.org**). A print version can also be requested from the American Cancer Society at **800-ACS-2345.**

The NCI provides treatment guidelines via its telephone information center (**800-4-CANCER**) and its Web site (**www.cancer.gov**). Detailed guidelines intended for use by cancer care professionals are also available at **www.cancer.gov.**

Questions to Ask

What Should You Ask Your Doctor About Colorectal Cancer?

It is important to have frank, open discussions with your doctor and other members of your cancer care team. They want to answer all your questions so that you can make informed treatment and life decisions. For instance, consider these questions:

- Where is my cancer located?
- Has my cancer spread beyond the **primary site**?
- What is the stage of my cancer and what does that mean in my case?
- What treatment choices do I have?
- What do you recommend and why?
- What risks or side effects are there to the treatments you suggest?
- What are the chances my cancer will come back with these treatment plans?
- What should I do to be ready for treatment?
- What can I do to reduce the side effects of treatment?

- Should I follow a special diet?
- What if I choose to do nothing?

In addition to these sample questions, be sure to write down some of your own. For instance, you might want more information about recovery times so you can plan your work schedule. Or you may want to ask about second opinions or about clinical trials for which you may qualify.

After Treatment

What Happens After Treatment for Colorectal Cancer?

Completing treatment can be both stressful and exciting. You will be relieved to finish treatment, yet it is hard not to worry about cancer coming back. This is a very common concern among those who have had cancer.

It may take awhile before your confidence in your own recovery begins to feel real and your fears are somewhat relieved. Even with no recurrences, people who have had cancer learn to live with uncertainty.

Follow-up Care

After your treatment is over, it is very important to keep all follow-up appointments. During these visits, your doctors will ask about symptoms, do physical exams, and may order blood tests or imaging tests such as CT scans or PET scans. Follow-up is needed to check for cancer recurrence or spread, as well as possible side effects of certain treatments. This is the time for you to discuss any concerns you might have with your cancer care team.

Almost any cancer treatment can have side effects. Some may last for a few weeks to several months, but others can be permanent. Do not hesitate to tell your cancer care team about any symptoms or side effects that bother you so they can help you manage them.

To some extent, the frequency of follow-up visits and tests will depend on the stage of your cancer and the likelihood of recurrence.

History and physical exam

Your doctor will likely recommend getting a history and physical exam every 3 to 6 months for the first 2 years after treatment, then every 6 months or so for the next few years. People who were treated for early-stage cancer may need less frequent exams.

Colonoscopy

In most cases, your doctor will recommend a colonoscopy within a year after surgery. If that test is normal, it should be repeated in 3 years. If that test is normal, then you can wait 5 years for your next colonoscopy.

Imaging tests

Whether your doctor recommends imaging tests will depend on the stage of your disease. CT scans may be done as frequently as once a year for those at higher risk of recurrence, especially in the first 2 years after surgery. Testing may be even more frequent in patients who have had tumors removed from their liver or lungs.

Blood tests for tumor markers

Carcinoembryonic antigen (CEA) and CA 19-9 are substances found in the blood of some people with colorectal cancer. Tests for 1 or both of these substances are sometimes useful if you have any symptoms that suggest the cancer has come back. Some doctors perform these tests every 3 to 6 months to detect recurrences before you have symptoms. Usually these are most important in the first 2 years after treatment, when most recurrences occur. If tumor marker levels start to rise, colonoscopy or imaging tests may be done to try to locate a recurrence.

For Patients with a Colostomy

If you have a colostomy, you may feel worried or isolated from normal activities. Whether your colostomy is temporary or permanent, an enterostomal therapist (a health care professional trained to help people with their colostomies) can teach you about the care of your colostomy. You can ask the American Cancer Society about programs offering information and support in your area. For more information, contact the American Cancer Society at **800-ACS-2345** and request the document *Colostomy: A Guide,* or look online: **www.cancer.org.**

Seeing a New Doctor

At some point after your cancer diagnosis and treatment, you may find yourself in the office of a new doctor. Your original doctor may have moved or retired, or you may have moved or changed doctors for some reason. It is important that you be able to give your new doctor the exact details of your diagnosis and treatment. Make sure you keep the following information handy:

- a copy of your pathology report(s) from any biopsy or surgery
- CT scan and MRI images on a transportable DVD
- if you had surgery, a copy of your operative report(s)
- if you were hospitalized, a copy of the discharge summary that doctors must prepare when patients are sent home
- if you had radiation therapy, a summary of the type and dose of radiation and when and where it was given
- if you had chemotherapy, a list of your drugs, drug doses, and when you took them

It is also important to keep medical insurance. Even though no one wants to think of their cancer coming back, it is always a possibility. If it happens, the last thing you want is to have to worry about paying for treatment.

Lifestyle Changes to Consider During and After Treatment

Having cancer and dealing with treatment can be time-consuming and emotionally draining, but it can also be a time to look at your life in new ways. Maybe you are thinking about how to improve your health over the long term. Some people even begin this process during cancer treatment.

Make Healthier Choices

Think about your life before you learned you had cancer. Were there things you did that might have made you less healthy? Maybe you drank too much alcohol, ate more than you needed, smoked, or didn't exercise very often. Emotionally, maybe you kept your feelings bottled up, or maybe you let stressful situations go on too long.

Now is not the time to feel guilty or to blame yourself. However, you can start making changes today that can have positive effects for the rest of your life. Not only will you feel better but you will also be healthier. What better time than now to take advantage of the motivation you have as a result of going through a life-changing experience like having cancer?

You can start by working on those things that you feel most concerned about. Get help with those that are harder for you. For instance, if you are thinking about quitting smoking and need help, call the American Cancer Society's Quitline℠ tobacco cessation program at **800-ACS-2345.**

Diet and Nutrition

Eating right can be a challenge for anyone, but it can get even tougher during and after cancer treatment. For instance, treatment often may change your sense of taste. Nausea can be a problem. You may lose your appetite for awhile and lose weight when you don't want to. On the other hand, some people gain weight even without eating more. This can be frustrating, too.

If you are losing weight or have taste problems during treatment, do the best you can with eating and remember that these problems usually improve over time. You may want to ask your cancer team for a referral to a dietitian, an expert in nutrition who can give you ideas on how to fight some of the side effects of your treatment. You may also find it helps to eat small portions every 2 to 3 hours until you feel better and can go back to a more normal schedule.

One of the best things you can do after treatment is to put healthy eating habits into place. You will be surprised at the long-term benefits of some simple changes, like increasing the variety of healthy foods you eat. Try to eat 5 or more servings of vegetables and fruits each day. Choose whole grain foods instead of white flour and sugars. Try to limit meats that are high in fat. Cut back on processed meats like hot dogs, bologna, and bacon. Get rid of them altogether if you can. If you drink alcohol, limit yourself to 1 or 2 drinks a day at the most. And don't forget to get some type of regular exercise. The combination of a good diet and regular exercise will help you maintain a healthy weight and keep you feeling more energetic.

Rest, Fatigue, Work, and Exercise

Fatigue is a very common symptom in people being treated for cancer. This is often not an ordinary type of tiredness but a bone-weary exhaustion that does not get better with rest. For some, this fatigue lasts a long time after treatment, and can discourage them from physical activity.

However, exercise can actually help you reduce fatigue. Studies have shown that patients who follow an exercise program tailored to their personal needs feel physically and emotionally improved and can cope better.

If you are ill and need to be on bed rest during treatment, it is normal to expect your fitness, endurance, and muscle strength to decline some. Physical therapy can help you maintain strength and range of motion in your muscles, which can help fight fatigue and the sense of depression that sometimes comes with feeling so tired.

Any program of physical activity should fit your own situation. An older person who has never exercised will not be able to take on the same amount of exercise as a 20-year-old who plays tennis 3 times a week. If you haven't exercised in a few years but can still get around, you may want to think about taking short walks.

Talk with your health care team before starting, and get their opinion about your exercise plans. Then, try to get an exercise buddy so that you're not doing it alone. Having family or friends involved when starting a new exercise program can give you that extra boost of support to keep you going when the push just is not there.

If you are very tired, though, you will need to balance activity with rest. It is okay to rest when you need to. It is really hard for some people to allow themselves to do that when they are used to working all day or taking care of a household. For more information, contact the American Cancer Society at **800-ACS-2345** and request the document *Cancer-Related Fatigue and Anemia Treatment Guidelines for Patients,* or look online: **www.cancer.org.**

Exercise can improve your physical and emotional health.

- It improves your cardiovascular (heart and circulation) fitness.
- It strengthens your muscles.
- It reduces fatigue.
- It lowers anxiety and depression.
- It makes you feel generally happier.
- It helps you feel better about yourself.

Any person who has been treated for colorectal cancer may also be at risk for a second colorectal cancer or even for other types of cancer. We know that exercise plays a role in preventing some types of cancer. The American Cancer Society, in its guidelines on physical activity for cancer prevention, recommends that adults take part in at least 1 physical activity for 30 minutes or more on 5 days or more of the week.

Can You Reduce Your Risk for Cancer Recurrence?

Most people want to know if there are things they can do to reduce their risk for cancer recurrence. Unfortunately, for most cancer there is little solid evidence that can guide people in this direction.

This does not mean that nothing will help—this is an area that has not been studied extensively. Most studies have looked at ways of preventing cancer in the first place, not preventing recurrences.

However, some studies have pointed to things people can do that *might* help reduce the risk of colorectal cancer returning.

Physical Activity

Two recent studies of people with earlier stage (I, II, or III) colorectal cancer showed that increasing recreational physical activity after diagnosis reduced the risk for death from colorectal cancer by as much as half. The level of activity needed to reduce risk was about 4 to 5 hours of brisk walking per week. More studies are needed to further define this possible benefit.

Diet

In a large study of patients with stage III colon cancer, those with the highest intakes of meat, fat, refined grains (sugars), and desserts were about 3 times more likely to have a recurrence than those who had the lowest intake of these foods. More research is needed to confirm these results and to determine which of these factors are most strongly linked to cancer recurrence.

How About Your Emotional Health?

Once your treatment ends, you may find yourself overwhelmed by emotions. This happens to a lot of people. You may have been going through so much during treatment that you could focus only on getting through your treatment.

Now you may find that you think about the potential of your own death, or the effect of your cancer on your family, friends, and career. You may also begin to re-evaluate your relationship with your spouse or partner. Unexpected issues may also cause concern—for instance, as you become healthier and have fewer doctor visits, you will see your cancer care team less often. That can be a source of anxiety for some.

This is an ideal time to seek emotional and social support. You need people you can turn to for strength and comfort. Support can come in many forms: family, friends, cancer support groups, church or spiritual groups, online support communities, or individual counselors.

Almost everyone who has been through cancer can benefit from getting some type of support. What is best for you depends on your situation and personality. Some people feel safe in peer-support groups or education groups. Others would rather talk in an informal setting, such as church. Others may feel more at ease talking one-on-one with a trusted friend or counselor. Whatever your source of strength or comfort, make sure you have a place to go with your concerns.

The cancer journey can feel very lonely. It is not necessary or realistic to go it all by yourself. Your friends and family may feel shut out if you decide not to include them. Let them in—and let in anyone else who you feel may help. If you aren't sure who can help, call your American Cancer Society at **800-ACS-2345,** and we can put you in touch with an appropriate group or resource.

You cannot change the fact that you have had cancer. What you can change is how you live the rest of your life—making healthy choices and feeling as well as possible, physically and emotionally.

What Happens If Treatment Is No Longer Working?

If cancer continues to grow after one kind of treatment, or if it returns, it is often possible to try another treatment plan that could still cure the cancer or shrink the tumors enough to help you live longer and feel better. On the other hand, when a person has undergone several medical treatments and the cancer has not been cured, the cancer can tend to become resistant to all treatment. At this time it is important to weigh the possible limited benefit of a new treatment against the possible downsides, including continued doctor visits and treatment side effects.

Everyone has his or her own way of looking at this decision. Some people may want to focus on remaining comfortable during the time they have.

This is likely to be the most difficult time in your battle with cancer—when you have tried every medical treatment within reason and it is just not working anymore. Although your doctor may offer you new treatment, you need to consider that, at some point, continuing treatment is not likely to improve your health or change your prognosis or survival.

If you want to continue treatment to fight your cancer for as long as you can, you still need to consider the odds of whether more treatment will have any benefit. In many cases, your doctor can estimate the response rate for the treatment you are considering. Some people are tempted to try more chemotherapy or radiation even when their doctors say that the odds of benefit are less than 1%. In this situation, you need to think about and understand your reasons for choosing this plan.

No matter what you decide to do, it is important that you be as comfortable as possible. Make sure you are asking for and getting treatment for any symptoms you might have, such as pain. This type of treatment is called **palliative treatment.**

Palliative treatment helps relieve these symptoms, but is not expected to cure the disease; its main purpose is to improve your **quality of life.** Sometimes, the treatments you get to control your symptoms are similar to the treatments used to treat cancer. For example, radiation therapy might be given to help relieve bone pain from bone metastasis, or chemotherapy might be given to help shrink a tumor and keep it from causing a bowel obstruction. This is not the same as receiving treatment to try to cure the cancer.

At some point, you may benefit from **hospice** care. Most of the time, this can be given at home. Your cancer may be causing symptoms or problems that need attention, and hospice focuses on your comfort. Receiving hospice care does not mean you cannot have treatment for the problems caused by your cancer or other health conditions. It just means that the focus of your care is on living life as fully as possible and feeling as well as you can at this difficult stage of your cancer.

Remember also that maintaining hope is important. Your hope for a cure may not be as bright, but there is still hope for good times with family and friends—times that are filled with happiness and meaning. In a way, pausing at this time in your cancer treatment is an opportunity to refocus on the most important things in your life. This is the time to do some things you have always wanted to do and to stop doing the things you no longer want to do.

Latest Research

What's New in Colorectal Cancer Research and Treatment?

Research is ongoing in the area of colorectal cancer. Scientists are looking for causes and ways to prevent colorectal cancer, as well as ways to improve treatments.

Genetics

Scientists are learning more about some of the inherited and acquired changes in DNA that cause cells of the colon and rectum to become cancerous. Recent discoveries of inherited genes that increase a person's risk of developing colorectal cancer are already being used in genetic tests to inform people who are at the highest risk.

Advances in understanding how these genes work are expected to eventually lead to new drugs and gene therapies to correct these gene problems. Early phases of gene therapy trials are already in progress.

Chemoprevention

Chemoprevention is the use of natural or manmade chemicals to lower a person's risk for cancer. Researchers are testing whether certain supplements, minerals (such as calcium), and vitamins (such as folic acid or vitamin D) can lower colorectal cancer risk.

Some studies have found that people who take multivitamins containing folic acid (also known as folate), vitamin D supplements, or a certain amount of calcium (through either diet or supplements) may have a lower risk of colorectal cancer than people who do not get enough of these nutrients. Research to clarify the possible benefits of these and other substances, such as selenium and curcumin, is now under way.

Although taking aspirin or some other nonsteroidal anti-inflammatory drugs (NSAIDs) is associated with a lower risk of colorectal cancer, these drugs can cause stomach ulcers and other side effects. For this reason, taking NSAIDs specifically for this purpose is not recommended for people at average risk of colorectal cancer.

NSAIDs, including sulindac and celecoxib (Celebrex), have been shown to reduce formation of adenomatous polyps in people with familial adenomatous polyposis (FAP). The FDA has approved celecoxib for reducing polyp formation in people with FAP. However, celecoxib may have side effects such as a potential increased heart risk. You should consult with your doctor before beginning regular use of aspirin or another NSAID.

Studies indicate that a diet high in fruits and vegetables may lower colorectal cancer risk, as well as the risk of several other diseases. This has not been completely proven by all studies. It is important that you eat enough servings—at least 5 a day. At this time, most experts recommend that people not take large doses of vitamins, minerals, or other agents unless they are part of a study or are under the advice and care of a doctor.

Earlier Detection

Colorectal cancer is much easier to treat effectively if it is found at a very early stage. Studies continue to look at the effectiveness of current colorectal cancer screening methods and assess new approaches to informing the public about the importance of being screened. Fewer than half of all Americans age 50 or older get colorectal cancer screening at all. If everyone were tested as recommended, tens of thousands of lives could be saved each year. The American Cancer Society and other public health organizations are working to increase awareness of colorectal cancer screening among the general public and health care professionals.

Meanwhile, new imaging and laboratory tests are also being developed and tested. Newer, more accurate ways to look for changes in the stool that might indicate colorectal cancer have been developed. These include tests that are better able to detect blood in the stool (fecal immunochemical tests) and tests that can detect changes in the DNA of cells in the stool. CT colonography (also known as virtual colonoscopy) is a special type of CT scan that can find colorectal polyps and cancer at least as accurately as a barium enema.

Treatment

Chemotherapy

Many clinical trials are testing new chemotherapy drugs or drugs that are now used against other types of cancer (such as cisplatin or gemcitabine). Other studies are looking at ways to combine drugs already known to be active against colorectal cancer, such as irinotecan or oxaliplatin, to improve their effectiveness. Newer studies are also looking at adding targeted therapies such as cetuximab or bevacizumab to chemotherapy as part of adjuvant therapy. Still other studies are testing the best ways to combine chemotherapy with radiation therapy and/or immunotherapy.

Targeted therapies

Several targeted therapies are already approved for treating colorectal cancer, including bevacizumab (Avastin), cetuximab (Erbitux), and panitumumab (Vectibix). Doctors continue to study the best way to give these drugs to make them as effective as possible.

Researchers are also studying dozens of new targeted therapies to increase the options for people with colorectal cancer. Some of these are monoclonal antibodies like the drugs listed above, while others are more like conventional drugs that are given in pill form.

Immunotherapy

Immunotherapy is aimed at enhancing the immune system's response to cancer. Researchers are studying several tumor vaccines to try to treat colorectal cancer or prevent it from coming back after treatment. Unlike vaccines that prevent infectious diseases, these vaccines are meant to boost the patient's immune reaction to fight colorectal cancer more effectively.

There are many types of vaccines being studied. For example, some vaccines involve removing some of the patient's own immune system cells (called dendritic cells) from the blood, exposing them in the laboratory to a substance that will make them attack cancer cells, and then putting them back into the body. At this time, such vaccines are available only in clinical trials.

Resources

Additional Resources

More Information from Your American Cancer Society

These related materials* may be viewed on our Web site or ordered from our toll-free number, **800-ACS-2345.**

After Diagnosis: A Guide for Patients and Families

ACS/NCCN Colon and Rectal Cancer: Treatment Guidelines for Patients (not available in Spanish)

Colostomy: A Guide

Nutrition for the Person with Cancer: A Guide for Patients and Families

Sexuality & Cancer: For the Man Who Has Cancer and His Partner

Sexuality & Cancer: For the Woman Who Has Cancer and Her Partner

Surgery

Understanding Chemotherapy: A Guide for Patients and Families

Understanding Radiation Therapy: A Guide for Patients and Families

---

*Most of these materials are also available in Spanish.

The following books are available from the American Cancer Society. Call us at **800-ACS-2345** to ask about costs or to place your order.

> *The American Cancer Society's Complete Guide to Colorectal Cancer*
>
> *Caregiving: A Step-By-Step Resource for Caring for the Person with Cancer at Home*

National Organizations and Web Sites*

In addition to the American Cancer Society, these are some other sources of patient information and support:

> American College of Gastroenterology
> Web site: **www.acg.gi.org**
>
> American Gastroenterological Association
> Telephone: **301-654-2055**
> Web site: **www.gastro.org**
>
> American Society of Colon and Rectal Surgeons
> Web site: **www.fascrs.org**
>
> Colon Cancer Alliance
> Toll-free number: **877-422-2030**
> Web site: **www.ccalliance.org**
>
> National Cancer Institute
> Toll-free number **800-4-CANCER** or
> **800-422-6237**; TTY: **800-332-8615**
> Web site: **www.cancer.gov**
>
> National Colorectal Cancer Research Alliance
> Web site: **www.eif.nccra.org**

No matter who you are, we can help. Contact us anytime, day or night, for information and support. Call us at **800-ACS-2345** or visit our Web site: **www.cancer.org.**

---

*Inclusion on this list does not imply endorsement by the American Cancer Society.

References

American Cancer Society. *Cancer Facts and Figures 2008.* Atlanta, GA: American Cancer Society: 2008.

American Joint Committee on Cancer. Colon and rectum. In: *AJCC Cancer Staging Manual. 6th ed.* New York, NY: Springer; 2002:113–124.

Balch GC, De Meo A, Guillem JG. Modern management of rectal cancer: a 2006 update. *World J Gastroenterol.* 2006;12(20):3186–3195.

Cole BF, Baron JA, Sandler RS, Haile RW, Ahnen DJ, Bresalier RS, McKeown-Eyssen G, Summers RW, Rothstein RI, Burke CA, Snover DC, Church TR, Allen JI, Robertson DJ, Beck GJ, Bond JH, Byers T, Mandel JS, Mott LA, Pearson LH, Barry EL, Rees JR, Marcon N, Saibil F, Ueland PM, Greenberg ER; Polyp Prevention Study Group. Folic acid for the prevention of colorectal adenomas: a randomized clinical trial. *JAMA.* 2007;297(21):2351–2359.

Gloeckler Ries LA, Reichman ME, Lewis DR, Edwards BK. Cancer survival and incidence from the Surveillance, Epidemiology, and End Results (SEER) program. *Oncologist.* 2003;8(6):541–552.

Hawk ET, Levin B. Colorectal cancer prevention. *J Clin Oncol.* 2005;23(2):378–391.

Hendriks YM, de Jong AE, Morreau H, Tops CM, Vasen HF, Wijnen JT, Breuning MH, Bröcker-Vriends AH. Diagnostic approach and management of Lynch syndrome (hereditary nonpolyposis colorectal carcinoma): a guide for clinicians. *CA Cancer J Clin.* 2006;56(4):213–225.

Levin B, Lieberman DA, McFarland B, Andrews KS, Brooks D, Bond J, Dash C, Giardiello FM, Glick S, Johnson D, Johnson CD, Levin TR, Pickhardt PJ, Rex DK, Smith RA, Thorson A, Winawer SJ; American Cancer Society Colorectal Cancer Advisory Group; US Multi-Society Task Force; American College of Radiology Colon Cancer

Committee. Screening and surveillance for the early detection of colorectal cancer and adenomatous polyps, 2008: a joint guideline from the American Cancer Society, the US Multi-Society Task Force on Colorectal Cancer, and the American College of Radiology. *Gastroenterology.* 2008;134(5):1570–1595.

Levin B, Brooks D, Smith RA, Stone A. Emerging technologies in screening for colorectal cancer. *CA Cancer J Clin.* 2003;53(1):44–55.

Libutti SK, Salz LB, Rustgi AK, Tepper JE. Cancer of the colon. In: DeVita VT, Hellman S, Rosenberg SA, eds. *Cancer: Principles and Practice of Oncology. 7th ed.* Philadelphia, PA: Lippincott Williams & Wilkins; 2005:1061–1109.

Libutti SK, Tepper JE , Salz LB, Rustgi AK. Cancer of the rectum. In: DeVita VT, Hellman S, Rosenberg SA, eds. *Cancer: Principles and Practice of Oncology. 7th ed.* Philadelphia, PA: Lippincott Williams & Wilkins; 2005:1110–1124.

Lindor NM, Petersen GM, Hadley DW, Kinney AY, Miesfeldt S, Lu KH, Lynch P, Burke W, Press N. Recommendations for the care of individuals with an inherited predisposition to Lynch syndrome: a systematic review. *JAMA.* 2006;296(12):1507–1517.

Locker GY, Lynch HT. Genetic factors and colorectal cancer in Ashkenazi Jews. *Fam Cancer.* 2004;3(3–4):215–221.

Lynch HT, de la Chapelle A. Hereditary colorectal cancer. *N Engl J Med.* 2003;348(10):919–932.

Meyerhardt JA, Giovannucci EL, Holmes MD, Chan AT, Chan JA, Colditz GA, Fuchs CS. Physical activity and survival after colorectal cancer diagnosis. *J Clin Oncol.* 2006;24(22):3527–3534.

Meyerhardt JA, Heseltine D, Niedzwiecki D, Hollis D, Saltz LB, Mayer RJ, Thomas J, Nelson H, Whittom R,

Hantel A, Schilsky RL, Fuchs CS. Impact of physical activity on cancer recurrence and survival in patients with stage III colon cancer: findings from CALGB 89803. *J Clin Oncol.* 2006;24(22):3535–3541.

Meyerhardt JA, Niedzwiecki D, Hollis D, Saltz LB, Hu FB, Mayer RJ, Nelson H, Whittom R, Hantel A, Thomas J, Fuchs CS. Association of dietary patterns with cancer recurrence and survival in patients with stage III colon cancer. *JAMA.* 2007;298(7):754–764.

National Cancer Institute. Colon Cancer Treatment (PDQ). 2007. Available at: www.cancer.gov/cancertopics/pdq/treatment/colon/healthprofessional. Accessed March 30, 2008.

National Cancer Institute. Rectal Cancer Treatment (PDQ). 2008. Available at: www.cancer.gov/cancertopics/pdq/treatment/rectal/healthprofessional. Accessed March 30, 2008.

National Cancer Institute. Surveillance Epidemiology and End Results (SEER) Cancer Statistics Review, 1975–2004. 2007. Available at: http://seer.cancer.gov/csr/1975_2004/sections.html. Accessed March 30, 2007.

National Comprehensive Cancer Network. NCCN Clinical Practice Guidelines in Oncology: Colon Cancer. V.1.2008. Available at: www.nccn.org/professionals/physician_gls/PDF/colon.pdf. Accessed March 30, 2008.

National Comprehensive Cancer Network. NCCN Clinical Practice Guidelines in Oncology: Rectal Cancer. V.1.2008. Available at: www.nccn.org/professionals/physician_gls/PDF/rectal.pdf. Accessed March 30, 2008.

Niederhuber JE, Cole CE, Grochow L, et al. Colon cancer. In: Abeloff MD, Armitage JO, Lichter AS, Niederhuber JE, Kastan MB, McKenna WG, eds. *Clinical Oncology.* 3rd ed. Philadelphia, PA: Elsevier; 2004:1877–1941.

O'Connell JB, Maggard MA, Ko CY. Colon cancer survival rates with the new American Joint Committee on Cancer Sixth Edition staging. *J Natl Cancer Inst*. 2004;96(19):1420–1425.

Regine WF, Hanna N, DeSimone P, Cohen AM. Cancer of the rectum. In: Abeloff MD, Armitage JO, Lichter AS, Niederhuber JE, Kastan MB, McKenna WG, eds. *Clinical Oncology*. 3rd ed. Philadelphia, PA: Elsevier; 2004:1942–1965.

Rex DK, Kahi CJ, Levin B, Smith RA, Bond JH, Brooks D, Burt RW, Byers T, Fletcher RH, Hyman N, Johnson D, Kirk L, Lieberman DA, Levin TR, O'Brien MJ, Simmang C, Thorson AG, Winawer SJ. Guidelines for colonoscopy surveillance after cancer resection: a consensus update by the American Cancer Society and U.S. Multi-Society Task Force on Colorectal Cancer. *CA Cancer J Clin*. 2006;56(3):160–167.

Schernhammer ES, Laden F, Speizer FE, Willett WC, Hunter DJ, Kawachi I, Fuchs CS, Colditz GA. Night-shift work and risk of colorectal cancer in the Nurses' Health Study. *J Natl Cancer Inst*. 2003;95(11):825–828.

Winawer SJ, Zauber AG, Fletcher RH, Stillman JS, O'Brien MJ, Levin B, Smith RA, Lieberman DA, Burt RW, Levin TR, Bond JH, Brooks D, Byers T, Hyman N, Kirk L, Thorson A, Simmang C, Johnson D, Rex DK. Guidelines for colonoscopy surveillance after polypectomy: a consensus update by the U.S. Multi-Society Task Force on Colorectal Cancer and the American Cancer Society. *CA Cancer J Clin*. 2006;56(3):143–159.

Glossary

abdomen (AB-duh-men): the part of the body between the chest and the pelvis. It contains the stomach (with the lower part of the esophagus), small and large intestines, liver, gallbladder, spleen, pancreas, and other organs. It is lined by a membrane called the peritoneum.

abdominoperineal (ab-dah-mih-no-pehr-ih-NEE-ul) resection: surgery in which the anus, rectum, and part of the colon are removed through an incision made in the abdomen. The end of the intestine is attached to an opening in the abdomen, called a stoma, and body waste is collected in a bag (appliance) outside of the body. Also called AP resection. *See also* colostomy.

adenocarcinoma (add-uh-no-kahr-si-NO-muh): cancer of the glandular cells, for example, those that line the inside of the colon and rectum.

adenoma (add-uh-NO-muh): a noncancerous tumor. *See* adenomatous polyp.

adenomatous polyp (add-uh-NO-muh-tus PAH-lip): a benign (noncancerous) growth of glandular cells, for example, those that line the inside of the colon or rectum. Also called adenoma. There are 3 types of colorectal adenomas: *tubular, villous,* and *tuberovillous.*

adhesions (ad-HEE-zhunz): scar tissue that forms after surgery. If it tightens, it may bind together organs that are normally separate. These can sometimes cause partial or total blockages of the intestine.

adjuvant (AJ-uh-vunt) therapy: treatment used in addition to the main treatment. It usually refers to hormone therapy, chemotherapy, radiation therapy, or immunotherapy added after surgery to increase the chances of curing the disease or prevent it from coming back.

AJCC staging system: *see* American Joint Committee on Cancer staging system.

alternative therapy (alternative medicine): an unproven medication or therapy that is recommended instead of standard (proven) therapy. Some alternative therapies have dangerous or even life-threatening side effects. With others, the main danger is that the patient may lose the opportunity to benefit from standard therapy. The American Cancer Society recommends that patients considering the use of any alternative or complementary therapies discuss them with their cancer care team. *See also* complementary therapy.

American Joint Committee on Cancer (AJCC) staging system: a system for describing the extent of a cancer's spread by using Roman numerals from 0 through IV. Also called the TNM system. *See also* staging.

Amsterdam criteria: a set of conditions common to people with hereditary nonpolyposis colon cancer (HNPCC). Only about 60% of people who meet all of the criteria actually have HNPCC, but people who meet the criteria may want to consider genetic testing for it. *Compare with* Bethesda Guidelines. *See also* hereditary nonpolyposis colon cancer.

anastomosis: the site where two structures are surgically joined together.

anemia (uh-NEEM-ee-uh): low red blood cell count.

anesthesia (an-es-THEE-zhuh): the loss of feeling or sensation as a result of drugs or gases. General anesthesia causes loss of consciousness (puts you to sleep). Local or regional anesthesia numbs only a certain area of the body.

angiogenesis (an-jee-o-JEN-uh-sis): the formation of new blood vessels. Some cancer treatments work by blocking angiogenesis, thus preventing blood from reaching the tumor.

angiogram: an x-ray of blood vessels. *See* angiography.

angiography (an-jee-AHG-ruh-fee): a test in which a contrast dye is injected directly into a blood vessel that goes to the area that is being studied. A series of x-ray images are taken to show surgeons the location of blood vessels around a tumor.

antibody: a protein produced by the body's immune system cells and released into the blood. Antibodies defend the body against foreign agents, such as bacteria. These agents contain certain substances called antigens. Each antibody works against a specific antigen. *See also* antigen.

antigen (AN-tuh-jen): a substance that causes the body's immune system to react. This reaction often involves production of antibodies. For example, the immune system's response to antigens that are part of bacteria and viruses helps people resist infections. Cancer cells have certain antigens that can be found by laboratory tests. Antigens are important in cancer diagnosis and in watching a patient's response to treatment. Other cancer cell antigens play a role in immune reactions that may help the body's resistance to cancer. *See also* antibody.

anus: the outlet of the digestive tract through which stool passes out of the body.

APC gene: a gene that slows the growth of cells in the body. Changes in this gene can cause familial adenomatous polyposis (FAP) and Gardner syndrome. People who have a mutation in this gene can develop hundreds of polyps in the colon. *See also* Gardner syndrome, familial adenomatous polyposis.

appendix: a small, close-ended tube attached to the cecum (the first part of the large intestine). *See* cecum.

AP resection: *see* abdominoperineal resection.

artery: a tube called a blood vessel that carries blood away from the heart to the tissues and organs in the body.

ascending colon: the first of the four sections of the colon. It extends upward on the right side of the abdomen.

Astler-Coller staging system: one of the staging systems for colorectal cancer. In this system, the letters A through D are used for the various stages.

barium sulfate: a chalky liquid used to outline the digestive tract for x-rays. It can be taken by mouth (as part of an upper GI series) or infused through the rectum as a barium enema (as part of a lower GI series).

benign: not cancer; not malignant.

Bethesda Guidelines: a set of conditions that are common to people with hereditary nonpolyposis colon cancer (HNPCC). Most people who meet these criteria actually do not have HNPCC, but may want to consider further testing for it. *Compare with* Amsterdam criteria. *See also* hereditary nonpolyposis colon cancer.

biopsy (BUY-op-see): the removal of a sample of tissue to see whether cancer cells are present. There are several kinds of biopsies. In an endoscopic biopsy, a small sample of tissue is removed by using instruments operated through a colonoscope. *See also* fine needle biopsy.

bowel: the intestine.

brachytherapy (brake-ee-THER-uh-pee): internal radiation treatment given by placing radioactive material directly into the tumor or close to it. Also called interstitial radiation therapy or seed implantation. *See* internal radiation. *Compare with* external beam radiation therapy.

CA 19-9: a tumor marker sometimes produced by colorectal, stomach, bile duct, and pancreatic cancers. It may also be produced in pancreatitis, liver disease, and other noncancerous conditions. *See* tumor marker.

cancer: cancer is not just one disease but a group of diseases. All forms of cancer cause cells in the body to change and grow out of control. Most types of cancer cells form a lump or mass called a tumor. The tumor can invade and destroy healthy tissue. Cells from the tumor can break away and travel to other parts of the body. There they can continue to grow. This spreading process is called metastasis. When cancer spreads, it is still named after the part of the body where it started. For example, if breast cancer spreads to the lungs, it is still called breast cancer, not lung cancer.

Some cancers, such as blood cancers, do not form a tumor. Not all tumors are cancer. A tumor that is not cancer is called benign. Benign tumors do not grow and spread the way cancer does. Benign tumors are usually not a threat to life. Another word for cancerous is malignant.

cancer care team: the group of health care professionals who work together to find, treat, and care for people with cancer. The cancer care team may include the following and others: primary care physicians, pathologists, oncology specialists (medical oncologist, radiation oncologist), surgeons (including surgical specialists such as urologists, gynecologists, neurosurgeons, etc.), nurses, oncology nurse specialists, and oncology social workers. Whether the team is linked formally or informally, there is usually one person who takes the job of coordinating the team.

cancer cell: a cell that divides and reproduces abnormally and has the potential to spread throughout the body, crowding out normal cells and tissue. *See also* metastasis.

carcinoembryonic antigen (kahr-si-no-em-bre-AHN-ik AN-tuh-jen) (CEA): a substance normally found in fetal tissue. If found in an adult, it may suggest that a cancer, especially one starting in the digestive system, may be present. Tests for this substance may help in finding out if a colorectal cancer has recurred after treatment. The test is not helpful for screening for colorectal cancer because of the large number of false positives and false negatives. *See* tumor marker, screening, false positive, false negative.

carcinoid (KAHR-sih-noid) tumors or carcinoids: tumors that develop from neuroendocrine cells, usually in the digestive tract, lung, or ovary. The cancer cells from these tumors release certain hormones into the bloodstream. In about 10% of people, the hormone levels are high enough to cause facial flushing, wheezing, diarrhea, a fast heartbeat, and other symptoms throughout the body.

carcinoma (kahr-si-NO-muh): any cancerous tumor that begins in the lining layer of organs. At least 80% of all cancers are carcinomas.

carcinoma in situ (kahr-si-NO-muh in SIGH-too): an early stage of cancer in which the tumor is confined to the organ where it first developed. The disease has not invaded other parts of the organ or spread to distant parts of the body. Most in situ carcinomas are highly curable. *See* in situ.

case manager: the member of a cancer care team, usually a nurse or oncology nurse specialist, who coordinates the patient's care throughout diagnosis, treatment, and recovery. The case manager provides guidance through the complex health care system by cutting through red tape, getting responses to questions, managing crises, and connecting the patient and family to needed resources.

catheter (CATH-uh-tur): a thin, flexible tube through which fluids enter or leave the body; e.g., a tube to drain urine.

CEA: *see* carcinoembryonic antigen.

cecum (SEE-kum): a pouch that connects the small intestine to the colon.

cell: the basic unit of which all living things are made. Cells replace themselves by splitting and forming new cells (mitosis). The processes that control the formation of new cells and the death of old cells are disrupted in cancer.

chemoprevention (key-mo-pre-VEN-shun): prevention or reversal of disease by using drugs, chemicals, vitamins, or minerals. Whereas this idea is not ready for widespread use, it is a very promising area of study.

chemotherapy (key-mo-THER-uh-pee): treatment with drugs to destroy cancer cells. Chemotherapy is often used, either alone or with surgery or radiation, to treat cancer that has spread or come back (recurred), or when there is a strong chance that it could recur.

clinical stage: an estimate of the extent of cancer based on physical exam, biopsy results, and imaging tests. *See also* pathologic staging, staging.

clinical trials: research studies to test new drugs or other treatments to compare current, standard treatments with others that may be better. Before a new treatment is used on people, it is studied in the laboratory. If laboratory studies suggest the treatment will work, the next step is to test its value for patients. These human studies are called clinical trials. The main questions the researchers want to answer are these:

- Does this treatment work?
- Does it work better than what we're now using?
- What side effects does it cause?
- Do the benefits outweigh the risks?
- Which patients are most likely to find this treatment helpful?

colectomy (ko-LEK-tuh-me): surgical removal of all (total colectomy) or part (partial colectomy or hemicolectomy) of the colon. *See also* laparoscopic-assisted colectomy.

colitis (ko-LIE-tis): a general term for inflammation of the large intestine (colon). Colitis is usually either intermittent or chronic (as in ulcerative colitis).

colon: the large intestine. The colon is a muscular tube about 5 feet long. It is divided into 4 sections: the ascending, transverse, descending, and sigmoid colon. It continues the process of absorbing water and mineral nutrients from food that was started in the small intestine.

colonoscope (ko-LAHN-oh-skope): a hollow, lighted tube that is slender and flexible, about the thickness of a finger. During a colonoscopy, it is inserted through the rectum up into the colon so the doctor can examine the inside of the colon. *See* colonoscopy.

colonoscopy (ko-lun-AHS-kuh-pee): a procedure that allows a doctor to see inside the large intestine to find polyps or cancer. During a colonoscopy, the colonoscope is inserted through the rectum up into the colon. A colonoscope is much longer than a sigmoidoscope and allows the doctor to see much more of the colon's lining. The colonoscope is connected to a video camera and video display monitor so the doctor can look closely at the inside of the colon.

colorectal cancer: since colon cancer and rectal cancer have many features in common, they are sometimes referred to together as colorectal cancer.

colostomy (kuh-LAHS-tuh-me): a procedure in which the end of the colon is attached to an opening created in the abdominal wall to get rid of body waste (stool). A colostomy is sometimes needed after surgery for cancer of the rectum. People with colon cancer sometimes have a temporary colostomy, but they rarely need a permanent one.

complementary therapy (complementary medicine): treatment used in addition to standard therapy. Some complementary therapies may help relieve certain symptoms of cancer, relieve side effects of standard cancer therapy, or improve a patient's sense of well-being. The American Cancer Society recommends that patients considering the use of any alternative or complementary therapies discuss these therapies with their cancer care team, since many of these treatments are unproven and some can be harmful. *See also* alternative therapy.

complete blood count (CBC): a test to check the level of red blood cells, white blood cells, and platelets in the blood.

computed tomography (to-MAHG-ruh-fee): an imaging test in which many x-rays are taken of a part of the body from different angles. These images are combined by a computer to produce cross-sectional pictures of internal organs. Except for the injection of a contrast dye (needed in some but not all cases), this is a painless procedure that can be done in an outpatient clinic. It is often referred to as "CT" or "CAT" scanning.

contrast solution: any material used in imaging studies, such as x-rays and MRI and CT scans, to help outline the body parts being examined. These solutions may be injected or ingested (drunk). Also called contrast dye, radiocontrast dye, radiocontrast medium. *See also* imaging tests.

control group: in research or clinical trials, the group that does not receive the treatment being tested. The group may get a placebo or sham treatment, or it may receive standard therapy. Also called the comparison group. *See also* clinical trials, randomized.

Crohn's (krohnz) disease: a type of chronic inflammatory bowel disease. In this condition, the small bowel or, less often, the colon is inflamed over a long period. This condition increases a person's risk for developing colon cancer, so starting colorectal cancer screening earlier and doing these tests more often is recommended. Also called Crohn's colitis. *See also* inflammatory bowel disease.

cryoablation (kry-oh-ab-LAY-shun): use of extreme cold to freeze and destroy cancer cells.

cryosurgery: *see* cryoablation.

CT colonography (koh-luhn-AHG-ruh-fee): *see* virtual colonoscopy.

CT–guided needle biopsy: a procedure that uses special x-rays to locate a mass, while the radiologist advances a biopsy needle toward it. The images are repeated until the doctor is sure the needle is in the tumor or mass. A small sample of tissue is then taken from the mass to be examined under a microscope. *See also* biopsy.

CT scan or **CAT scan:** *see* computed tomography.

curative treatment: treatment aimed at producing a cure. *Compare with* palliative treatment.

deoxyribonucleic (dee-ox-ee-rie-bo-noo-KLAY-ik) acid: see DNA.

descending colon: the third section of the colon; it continues downward on the left side of the abdomen.

detection: finding disease. Early detection means that the disease is found at an early stage, before it has grown large or spread to other sites. Note: many forms of cancer can reach an advanced stage without causing symptoms.

diagnosis: identifying a disease by its signs or symptoms and by using imaging procedures and laboratory findings. For some types of cancer, the earlier a diagnosis is made, the better the chance for long-term survival.

digestive system: the collection of organs (also called the gastrointestinal tract, or GI tract) that processes food for energy and rids the body of solid waste matter.

digital rectal examination (DRE): an exam during which the doctor inserts a lubricated, gloved finger into the rectum to feel for anything abnormal. This simple test, which is not painful, can be used to detect many rectal cancers.

double-contrast barium enema (DCBE): a method used to help diagnose colorectal cancer. Barium sulfate, a chalky substance, is infused through the rectum to partially fill and open up the colon. When the colon is about half-full of barium, air is inserted to cause the colon to expand. This allows x-ray films to show abnormalities of the colon. Also called barium enema with air contrast or air-contrast barium enema.

DNA: deoxyribonucleic acid. DNA is the genetic "blueprint" found in the nucleus of each cell. It holds genetic information on cell growth, division, and function.

DRE: *see* digital rectal examination.

Dukes staging system: one of the staging systems for colorectal cancer, it uses the letters A through C.

dysplasia (dis-PLAY-zhuh): abnormal changes of groups in cells that may lead to cancer.

endorectal MRI: an MRI done from inside the rectum. *See also* magnetic resonance imaging.

enema: the injection of a liquid through the anus into the rectum.

enterostomal (en-tur-oh-STOH-mul) therapist: a health professional, often a nurse, who teaches people how to care for ostomies (surgically created openings such as a colostomy) and other wounds.

epidermal growth factor receptor (EGFR): a protein found on the surface of some cells. Epidermal growth factor binds to EGFR and causes the cells to divide. EGFR is found in high levels on the surface of many cancer cells.

esophagus: the tube connecting the throat to the stomach.

ethanol (alcohol) ablation: *see* percutaneous ethanol injection.

external beam radiation therapy (EBRT): radiation that is focused from a source outside the body on the area affected by the cancer. It is much like getting a diagnostic x-ray, but for a longer period. *Compare with* brachytherapy, internal radiation therapy.

false negative: test result implying a condition does not exist when, in fact, it does.

false positive: test result implying a condition exists when, in fact, it does not.

familial adenomatous polyposis (fuh-MIL-ee-uhl add-uh-NO-muh-tus pahl-ih-POH-sis) (FAP): an inherited condition that is a risk factor for colorectal cancer. People with this syndrome typically develop hundreds of polyps in the colon and rectum. Usually one or more of these polyps becomes cancerous if preventive surgery is not done.

fecal immunochemical (FEE-kuhl im-you-no-KIM-uh-kuhl) test (FIT): a newer test to detect "hidden" blood in the stool, which could be a sign of cancer. The test is not affected by vitamins or foods, though it still requires 2 or 3 specimens. Also called immunochemical fecal occult blood test. *See also* fecal occult blood test, false positive, screening.

fecal occult blood test (FOBT): a test for "hidden" blood in the feces (stool). The presence of such blood could be a sign of cancer. *See also* fecal immunochemical test, guaiac test, screening.

feces: solid waste matter; stool.

FDA: *see* U.S. Food and Drug Administration.

fiber: dietary fiber includes a wide variety of plant carbohydrates that are not digested by humans. Fibers are classified as "soluble" (like oat bran) and "insoluble" (like wheat bran). Soluble fiber helps to reduce blood cholesterol, thereby lowering the risk of heart disease. Good sources of fiber are beans, vegetables, whole grains, and fruits. Links between fiber and cancer risk are inconclusive. Eating these foods is still recommended because they have other health benefits and contain other substances that can help prevent cancer.

fine needle biopsy: a procedure in which a thin needle is used to draw up samples for examination under a microscope. Fine needle biopsy is not generally used for biopsies of a colorectal tumor, but is often used to take samples of masses in the liver or other organs that might be colorectal cancer metastases. *See also* biopsy.

first-degree relative: a parent, sibling, or child. *Compare with* second-degree relative.

first-line treatment: the first treatment for a disease. *Compare with* second-line treatment.

five (5)-year survival rate: the percentage of people with a given cancer who are expected to survive 5 years or longer with the disease. Five-year survival rates have some drawbacks. Although the rates are based on the most recent information available, they may include data from patients treated several years earlier. Advances in cancer treatment often occur quickly. Five-year survival rates, while statistically valid, may not reflect these advances. They should not be seen as a predictor in an individual case. *See also* relative five (5)-year survival rate.

flexible sigmoidoscopy (sig-moi-DAHS-kuh-pee): a procedure in which a doctor can look into the rectum and the descending portion of the colon for polyps or other abnormalities. During flexible sigmoidoscopy, the doctor inserts a flexible tube called a sigmoidoscope through the rectum and into the colon to look for cancer or polyps. The sigmoidoscope is connected to a video camera and video display monitor so the doctor can look closely at the inside of the colon. This test may be somewhat uncomfortable, but it should not be painful. *See also* sigmoidoscope.

folic acid: a B vitamin found in green plants, fruit, liver, and other foods. Folic acid is being studied as a possible cancer prevention agent. Also called folate.

Gardner syndrome: like familial adenomatous polyposis, Gardner syndrome is an inherited condition that results in polyps that develop at a young age and often lead to cancer. It can also cause benign (noncancerous) tumors of the skin, soft connective tissue, and bones.

gastroenterologist (gas-troh-en-tur-AHL-uh-jist): a doctor who specializes in diseases of the digestive (gastrointestinal) tract.

gastrointestinal stromal (gas-tro-en-TES-tih-nuhl STROH-muhl) tumors (GISTs): rare tumors of the connective tissue in the wall of the small intestine, colon, and rectum.

gastrointestinal (GI) tract: the digestive tract. It consists of those organs and structures that process food to be used for energy.

gene: a segment of DNA that contains information on hereditary characteristics such as hair color, eye color, and height, as well as susceptibility to certain diseases. *See also* DNA.

genetic counseling: the process of counseling people who may have a gene that makes them more susceptible to cancer. The purpose of the counseling is to help them decide whether they wish to be tested, to explore what the genetic test results might mean, and to support them before and after the test.

genetic counselor: a specially trained health professional who helps people as they consider genetic testing, as they adjust to the test results, and as they consider whatever screening and preventive measures are best for them.

genetic risk factor: a risk factor that is inherited from a parent. A risk factor is anything that increases a person's chance of getting a disease such as cancer. Risk factors can be lifestyle-related or environmental, or genetic (inherited). Having a risk factor, or several risk factors, does not mean that a person will get the disease. Most cancers are not caused by genetic risk factors. If a patient has several family members with cancer, however, genetic testing may be considered. *See also* risk factor.

genetic testing: tests performed to see if a person has certain gene changes known to increase cancer risk. Such testing is not recommended for everyone, rather for those with specific types of family history. Genetic counseling should be part of the process.

grade: the grade of a cancer reflects how abnormal it looks under the microscope. There are several grading systems for different types of cancers. Each grading system divides cancer into those with the greatest abnormality, the least abnormality, and those in between.

Grading is done by a pathologist who examines the tissue from the biopsy. It is important because cancers with more abnormal-appearing cells tend to grow and spread more quickly and have a worse prognosis (outlook). *See also* pathologist, prognosis.

guaiac (GWI-ack) test: another name for a fecal occult blood test (FOBT). Guaiac is the substance that can interact with and detect very small amounts of blood in the stool. Hemoccult is a brand of guaiac test.

helical (HEEL-ih-kuhl) CT or helical computed tomography: A detailed picture of the inside of the body, created by a computer linked to an x-ray machine. The CT machine rotates around the patient's body in a spiral path. Also called spiral CT. *See also* computed tomography, spiral CT.

hemicolectomy: surgical removal of part of the colon. Also called partial colectomy.

hemoglobin: the iron-containing substance inside red blood cells.

hepatic arterial infusion (huh-PAT-ik ar-TEER-ee-uhl in-FYOO-zhun): a procedure to deliver chemotherapy directly to the liver. Catheters are put into an artery that leads directly to the liver, and drugs are given through the catheters.

hepatic artery: the major blood vessel that carries blood to the liver. *See also* hepatic arterial infusion, hepatic artery embolization.

hepatic (huh-PAT-ik) artery embolization (em-buh-lie-ZAY-shun): a type of treatment for tumors in the liver that cannot be removed. It reduces the blood supply to the cancer by the injection of materials to plug up the hepatic artery, which supplies blood to the tumor.

hereditary nonpolyposis (non-pahl-ih-POH-sis) colon cancer (HNPCC): an inherited condition that increases a person's risk for developing colorectal cancer. People with this condition tend to develop cancer at a young age without first having many polyps. *See also* Lynch syndrome.

hormone replacement therapy: a therapy in which hormones are given to women after menopause to replace the hormones no longer produced by the body. Also called HRT.

hospice: a special kind of care for people in the final phase of illness, their families, and caregivers. The care may take place in the patient's home or in a home-like facility.

hyperplastic polyp: a common benign growth in the colon lining. Hyperplastic polyps are rarely a risk factor for colorectal cancer.

ileostomy (il-ee-AHS-tuh-me): an operation in which the end of the small intestine, the ileum, is attached to an opening in the abdominal wall. The contents of the intestine, unformed stool, are expelled through this opening into a bag called an appliance.

imaging tests: methods used to produce pictures of internal body structures. Some imaging methods used to help diagnose or stage cancer are x-rays, CT scans, magnetic resonance imaging (MRI), and ultrasound.

immunotherapy (im-you-no-THER-uh-pee): treatments that promote or support the body's immune system response to a disease such as cancer.

inflammatory bowel disease: a chronic condition (either ulcerative colitis or Crohn's disease) in which the colon is inflamed over a long period and may have ulcers in its lining, and which increases a person's risk of colorectal cancer.

inflammatory polyp: a type of polyp that can be associated with ulcerative colitis. *See* ulcerative colitis.

informed consent: a legal document that explains a course of treatment, the risks, benefits, and possible alternatives; the process by which patients agree to treatment.

in situ (in SIGH-too): in place; localized and confined to one area. A very early stage of cancer.

internal radiation therapy: treatment involving implantation of a radioactive substance. *See* brachytherapy. *Compare with* external beam radiation therapy.

intestines: the part of the digestive tract from the end of the stomach (pylorus) to the anus, which absorbs nutrients and water from food into the bloodstream. It includes the small intestine and the large intestine.

intravenous (in-tra-VEEN-us) (IV) line: a method of supplying fluids and medications by using a needle or a thin tube inserted in a vein.

irritable bowel syndrome: a condition marked by changes in bowel habits, abdominal pain, and bloating or gas. Irritable bowel syndrome does not increase risk of colorectal cancer. *Compare with* inflammatory bowel disease.

laparoscope (LAP-uh-ro-skope): a long, slender tube inserted into the abdomen through a very small incision. Surgeons with experience in laparoscopy can do some types of surgery for colorectal cancer using special surgical instruments operated through the laparoscope. *See also* laparoscopy.

laparoscopic-assisted colectomy (lap-uh-ro-SKAHP-ik assisted ko-LEK-tuh-me): surgery done with the aid of a laparoscope to remove al or part of the colon. *See also* laparoscopy, laparoscope, colectomy.

laparoscopy (lap-uh-RAHS-kuh-pee): examination of the abdominal cavity with an instrument called a laparoscope.

large intestine: *see* colon.

laxative: a substance that stimulates bowel movements.

linear accelerator: a machine used in radiation therapy to treat cancer. It gives off gamma rays and electron beams. This is called external beam radiation therapy.

liver: a large organ in the upper abdomen. The liver is one of the most common sites of colorectal cancer metastases.

local excision (eck-SIH-zhun): surgery to remove small superficial (surface) cancers or polyps.

local or localized cancer: a cancer that is confined to the organ where it started; that is, it has not spread to distant parts of the body.

lower GI series: series of x-rays of the intestines taken after a barium enema is given.

lymph (limf): clear fluid that flows through the lymphatic vessels and contains cells known as lymphocytes. These cells are important in fighting infections and may also have a role in fighting cancer. *See also* lymphatic system, lymph nodes, lymphocyte, lymphadenectomy.

lymph nodes: small bean-shaped collections of immune system tissue such as lymphocytes, found along lymphatic vessels. They remove cell waste, germs, and other harmful substances from lymph. They help fight infections and also have a role in fighting cancer, although cancers sometimes spread through lymph nodes. Also called lymph glands. *See also* lymph, lymphatic system, lymphadenectomy.

lymphadenectomy (lim-fad-uh-NECK-tuh-me): surgical removal of one or more lymph nodes. After removal, the lymph nodes are examined by microscope to see if cancer has spread. Also called lymph node dissection. *See also* lymphatic system, lymph, lymph nodes, lymphocyte.

lymphatic system: a network of tissues and organs (including lymph nodes, spleen, thymus, and bone marrow) that produce and store lymphocytes (cells that fight infection) and the channels that carry the lymph fluid. The lymphatic system is an important part of the body's immune system, as its function is to fight infection. Invasive cancers sometimes penetrate the lymphatic vessels (channels) and spread (metastasize) to lymph nodes. *See also* lymph, lymph nodes, lymphocyte, lymphadenectomy.

lymphatic vessel: a thin vessel that carries lymph and white blood cells. *See also* lymph, lymphatic system.

lymphocyte (LIM-fo-sight): a type of white blood cell that helps the body fight infection.

lymphoma (lim-FOAM-uh): a cancer of the lymphatic system. Lymphoma involves a type of white blood cells called lymphocytes. The 2 main types of lymphoma are Hodgkin disease and non-Hodgkin lymphoma. The treatment methods for these 2 types of lymphomas are very different. *See* lymphatic system.

Lynch syndrome: an inherited disorder in which a person is at increased risk of developing colorectal cancer, usually before the age of 50. Also called hereditary nonpolyposis colon cancer or HNPCC. *See* hereditary nonpolyposis colon cancer.

magnetic resonance imaging (MRI): a method of taking pictures of the inside of the body. Instead of using x-rays, MRI uses a powerful magnet to send radio waves through the body. The images appear on a computer screen, as well as on film. Like x-rays, the procedure is physically painless, but some people may feel confined inside the MRI machine.

malignant: cancerous.

malignant tumor: a mass of cancer cells that may invade surrounding tissues or spread (metastasize) to distant sites in the body. *See also* tumor, metastasis.

medical oncologist: a doctor who is specially trained to diagnose cancer and treat it with chemotherapy and other drugs.

metastasis (meh-TAS-teh-sis): cancer cells that have spread to one or more sites elsewhere in the body, often by way of the lymphatic system or bloodstream. Regional metastasis is cancer that has spread to the lymph nodes, tissues, or organs close to the primary site. Distant metastasis is cancer that has spread to organs or tissues that are farther away (such as when colon cancer spreads to the lungs or liver). The plural of this word is metastases. *See also* primary site, lymph nodes, lymphatic system, local or localized cancer, regional involvement, or regional spread.

metastasize (meh-TAS-tuh-size): the spread of cancer cells to one or more sites elsewhere in the body, often by way of the lymphatic system or bloodstream. *See also* metastasis, lymphatic system.

metastatic (met-uh-STAT-ick) cancer: a way to describe cancer that has spread from the primary site (where it started) to other structures or organs, nearby or far away (distant). *See also* primary site, metastasis.

monoclonal (mahn-oh-KLOHN-uhl) antibody: a type of antibody manufactured in the laboratory that is designed to lock onto specific antigens. Antigens are substances that can be recognized by the immune system. Monoclonal antibodies that have been attached to chemotherapy drugs or radioactive substances are being studied for their potential to seek out antigens unique to cancer cells and deliver these treatments directly to the cancer, thus killing the cancer cells and not harming healthy tissue. Monoclonal antibodies are also often used to help detect and classify cancer cells under a microscope. Other studies are being done to see if radioactive atoms attached to monoclonal antibodies can be used in imaging tests to detect and locate small groups of cancer cells. *See* antibody, antigen.

MRI: *see* magnetic resonance imaging.

mucinous carcinoma (MYOO-sih-nuhs kahr-si-NO-muh): a type of adenocarcinoma that is formed by cancer cells that produce large amounts of mucus.

mucosa: mucous membrane; the innermost lining layer of the colon and rectum. *See also* submucosa.

mucus: the thick fluid secreted by mucous membranes and glands.

muscularis mucosa: a thin layer of muscle under the mucosa. *See* mucosa.

muscularis propria: the thick layer of muscle in the colon and rectum that helps push the contents of the intestines through.

neoadjuvant (nee-oh-AJ-oo-vunt) therapy: treatment given before the main treatment. *Compare with* adjuvant therapy.

nonsteroidal anti-inflammatory drug: a drug that decreases fever, swelling, pain, and redness. Also called NSAID.

NSAID: see nonsteroidal anti-inflammatory drug.

nurse practitioner: a registered nurse with a master's or doctoral degree. Licensed nurse practitioners diagnose and manage illness and disease, usually working closely with a doctor. In many states, they may prescribe medications.

oncogenes: genes that promote cell growth and multi-plication. These genes are normally present in all cells. But oncogenes may undergo changes that activate them, causing cells to grow too quickly and form tumors.

oncologist (on-CAHL-uh-jist): a doctor with special training in the diagnosis and treatment of cancer.

oncology: the branch of medicine concerned with the diagnosis and treatment of cancer.

oncology clinical nurse specialist: a registered nurse with a master's degree in oncology who specializes in the care of cancer patients. Oncology nurse specialists may prepare and administer treatments, monitor patients, prescribe and provide supportive care, and teach and counsel patients and their families.

oncology social worker: a person with a master's degree in social work who is an expert in coordinating and providing non-medical care to patients. The oncology social worker provides counseling and assistance to people with cancer and their families, especially in dealing with the non-medical issues that can result from cancer, such as financial problems, housing (when treatments must be taken at a facility away from home), and child care.

osteoporosis (os-tee-oh-puh-ROH-sis): thinning of bone tissue, resulting in less bone mass and weaker bones. Osteoporosis can cause pain, deformity (especially of the spine), and broken bones. This condition is common among postmenopausal women.

p53: a protein that is mutated in more than 50% of tumors. The normal (not mutated) form of p53 keeps the cell from entering the cell division cycle. It has also been found to bring about cell death (apoptosis) after DNA damage.

palliative (PAL-ee-uh-tiv) treatment: treatment that relieves symptoms, such as pain, but is not expected to cure the disease. Its main purpose is to improve the patient's quality of life. Sometimes chemotherapy and radiation are used as palliative treatments.

pancolitis (pan-koh-LIE-tis): inflammation of the entire colon. *See also* colitis.

pathologic stage: an estimate of the extent of cancer by direct study of the samples removed during surgery. *See also* clinical stage, staging.

pathologist (path-AHL-o-jist): a doctor who specializes in diagnosis and classification of diseases by laboratory tests such as examining cells under a microscope. The pathologist determines whether a tumor is benign or cancerous and, if cancerous, the exact cell type and grade.

pelvic exenteration (ek-sen-tur-AY-shun): surgery to remove the organs in the pelvis.

percutaneous (pur-kyoo-TAY-nee-us) ethanol injection: injection of alcohol directly into a tumor to kill cancerous cells. Also called ethanol (alcohol) ablation.

peritoneum (pehr-ih-to-NEE-um): the membrane that lines the abdomen and covers most of its organs. Peritoneal cavity refers to the area enclosed by the peritoneum.

PET scan: *see* positron emission tomography.

Peutz-Jeghers (pootz JAY-gerz) syndrome: an inherited condition in which polyps form in the intestine. Dark freckles may also appear on the mouth and fingers. Having the disorder increases a person's risk for many types of cancer, including colorectal cancer. Also called PJS.

polyp: a growth from a mucous membrane commonly found in organs such as the rectum, the colon, or other organs. Some polyps may be precancerous or may contain cancer cells.

polypectomy (pahl-ih-PEK-tuh-mee): surgery to remove a polyp.

portal vein: a vein that carries blood from the digestive organs, spleen, pancreas, and gallbladder to the liver.

positron emission tomography (PAHS-ih-trahn ee-MISH-uhn toh-MAHG-ruh-fee) (PET): a PET scan creates an image of the body (or of biochemical events) after the injection of a very low dose of a radioactive form of a substance such as glucose (sugar). The scan computes the rate at which the tumor is using the sugar. In general, high-grade tumors use more sugar than normal and low-grade tumors use less. PET scans are especially useful in taking images of the brain, although they are becoming more widely used to find the spread of cancer of the breast, colon, rectum, ovary, or lung. PET scans may also be used to see how well the tumor is responding to treatment.

precancerous: changes in cells that may, but do not always, become cancer.

primary site: the place where cancer begins. Primary cancer is usually named after the organ in which it starts. For example, cancer that starts in the colon is always colon cancer even if it spreads (metastasizes) to other organs such as the liver or lungs.

prognosis (prog-NO-sis): a prediction of the course of disease; the outlook for the chances of survival.

protocol: a formal outline or plan, such as a description of what treatments a patient will receive and exactly when each should be given. *See also* regimen.

quality of life: overall enjoyment of life, which includes a person's sense of well-being and ability to do the things that are important to him or her.

radiation oncologist: a doctor who specializes in using radiation to treat cancer.

radiation proctitis: a possible side effect of radiation therapy, involving inflammation of the rectum and anus. Problems can include pain, bowel frequency, bowel urgency, bleeding, chronic burning, or rectal leakage.

radiation therapy: treatment with high-energy rays (such as x-rays) to kill or shrink cancer cells. The radiation may come from outside of the body (external radiation) or from radioactive materials placed directly in the tumor (brachytherapy or internal radiation). Radiation therapy may be used as the main treatment for a cancer, to reduce the size of a cancer before surgery, or to destroy any remaining cancer cells after surgery. In advanced cancer cases, it may also be used as palliative treatment. *See also* external beam radiation therapy, brachytherapy, palliative treatment.

radiofrequency ablation (RAY-dee-oh-free-kwin-see uh-BLAY-shun): treatment that uses electric current to destroy abnormal tissues. A thin, needle-like probe is guided into the tumor by ultrasound or CT scan. The probe releases a high-frequency current that heats and destroys cancer cells.

radiologist: a doctor with special training in diagnosis of diseases by interpreting x-rays and other types of diagnostic imaging tests; for example, CT and MRI scans.

randomized or randomization: a process used in clinical trials that uses chance to assign participants to different groups that compare treatments. Randomization means that each person has an equal chance of being in the treatment and comparison groups. This helps reduce the chance of bias in the results that might happen, if, for example, the healthiest people all were assigned to a particular treatment group. *See also* control group, clinical trials.

rectum: the lower part of the large intestine, just above the anus.

recurrence: the return of cancer after treatment. Local recurrence means that the cancer has come back at the same place as the original cancer. Regional recurrence means that the cancer has come back after treatment in the lymph nodes near the primary site. Distant recurrence, also known as metastatic recurrence, is when cancer metastasizes *after* treatment to distant organs or tissues (such as the lungs, liver, bone marrow, or brain). *See also* primary site, metastasis, metastasize, relapse.

red blood cells: blood cells that contain hemoglobin, the substance that carries oxygen to all of the cells of the body. *See also* anemia.

regimen (REH-juh-men): a strict, regulated plan (such as diet, exercise, or medication schedule) designed to reach certain goals. In cancer treatment, a plan to treat cancer.

regional involvement: the spread of cancer from its original site to nearby areas such as lymph nodes, but not to distant sites.

regional recurrence or regional spread: the spread of cancer from its original site to nearby areas such as lymph nodes, but not to distant sites. *See also* metastasis, recurrence.

relapse: reappearance of cancer after a disease-free period. *See also* recurrence.

relative five (5)-year survival rate: the percentage of people with a certain cancer who have not died of it within 5 years. This number is different from the 5-year survival rate in that it does not include people who have died of unrelated causes.

remission: complete or partial disappearance of the signs and symptoms of cancer in response to treatment; the period during which a disease is under control. A remission may not be a cure.

resection: surgery to remove part or all of an organ or other structure.

risk factor: anything that affects a person's chance of getting a disease such as cancer. Different cancers have different risk factors. For example, unprotected exposure to strong sunlight is a risk factor for skin cancer; smoking is a risk factor for lung, mouth, larynx, and other cancers. Some risk factors, such as smoking, can be controlled. Others, like a person's age, can't be changed.

screening: the search for disease, such as cancer, in people without symptoms. For example, screening measures recommended by the American Cancer Society for colorectal cancer include one of the following: flexible sigmoidoscopy; fecal occult blood test; flexible sigmoidoscopy plus fecal occult blood test; colonoscopy; or double contrast barium enema. Screening may also refer to coordinated programs in large populations.

second-degree relative: an aunt, uncle, grandparent, grandchild, niece, nephew, or half-sibling. *Compare with* first-degree relative.

second-line treatment: treatment that is given when the first-line treatment does not work or stops working.

segmental resection: surgery in which the cancer and a length of normal colon on either side of the cancer, as well as the nearby lymph nodes, are removed. The remaining sections of the colon are then reattached.

serosa (seer-OH-suh): a membrane lining the organs and body cavities of the chest and abdomen. *See also* subserosa.

side effects: unwanted effects of treatment, such as hair loss caused by chemotherapy and fatigue caused by radiation therapy.

sigmoid colon: the fourth section of the colon. It is known as the sigmoid colon because of its S-shape. The sigmoid colon attaches to the rectum, which in turn connects to the anus, the opening where waste matter passes out of the body.

sigmoidoscope (sig-MOI-do-skope): a slender, flexible, hollow, lighted tube about the thickness of a finger. It is inserted through the rectum up into the colon during a flexible sigmoidoscopy. This allows the doctor to look for cancer or for polyps inside the rectum and part of the colon. *See* flexible sigmoidoscopy.

sigmoidoscopy: *see* flexible sigmoidoscopy.

sign: an observable physical change caused by an illness. *Compare with* symptom.

small intestine: the longest section of the GI tract. It breaks down food and absorbs most of the nutrients. The small intestine leads into the colon.

sphincter: a ring-shaped muscle that controls the restriction and expansion of a body passage. The anal sphincter controls the opening of the anus. *See* anus.

spiral CT: a special scanner that takes cross-sectional pictures around the body. *See also* computed tomography, helical CT.

stage: the extent of a cancer in the body. *See* staging.

staging: the process of finding out whether cancer has spread and if so, how far. There is more than one system for staging colorectal cancer, including the AJCC/TNM, Dukes, and Astler-Coller systems.

The TNM system, which is used most often, gives 3 key pieces of information:

- T refers to the size of the tumor
- N describes how far the cancer has spread to nearby lymph nodes
- M shows whether the cancer has spread (metastasized) to other organs of the body

Letters or numbers after the T, N, and M give more details about each of these factors. To make this information more clear, the TNM descriptions can be grouped together into a simpler set of stages, labeled with Roman numerals (usually from I to IV). In general, the lower the number, the less the cancer has spread. A higher number means a more serious cancer.

The 2 types of staging are clinical staging and pathologic staging. *See also* clinical stage, pathologic stage.

standard therapy: the most commonly used and widely accepted form of treatment for a disease.

stoma: an opening, especially an opening made by surgery to allow elimination of body waste. *See also* colostomy, ileostomy, urostomy.

stomach: one of the principal organs of digestion, located between the esophagus and small intestine.

stool: solid waste matter; feces.

stool DNA test: a test in which a stool sample is examined for DNA from cancer cells.

submucosa: the layer of tissue beneath the mucosa. *See* mucosa.

subserosa: the layer of tissue beneath the serosa. *See* serosa.

symptom: a change in the body caused by an illness, as described by the person experiencing it. *Compare with* sign.

systemic therapy: treatment that reaches and affects cells throughout the entire body; for example, chemotherapy.

targeted therapy: treatment that attacks some part of cancer cells that make them different from normal cells, as opposed to treatment that harms all cells. Targeted therapy tends to have fewer side effects than some standard treatments such as chemotherapy.

tissue: a collection of cells, united to perform a particular function in the body.

TNM staging system: *see* staging.

total colon exam (TCE): an exam that looks at the entire large intestine, such as colonoscopy or double-contrast barium enema.

transverse colon: the second section of the colon. It is called the transverse colon because it goes across the body from the right to the left side.

tumor: an abnormal lump or mass of tissue. Tumors can be benign (noncancerous) or malignant (cancerous).

tumor marker: a substance produced by cancer cells and sometimes normal cells. Tumor markers are not very useful for cancer screening because other body tissues not related to a cancer can produce the substance. Tumor markers may be very useful in monitoring for response to treatment when a cancer is diagnosed or for a recurrence. Tumor markers include CA 125 (ovarian cancer), CEA (GI tract cancers), and PSA (prostate cancer).

tumor suppressor genes: genes that slow down cell division or cause cells to die at the appropriate time. Alterations of these genes can lead to too much cell growth and development of cancer.

tumor vaccine: an experimental treatment for cancer, in which a patient's own cancer cells are injected into the blood of the patient, or mixed with the patient's white blood cells in the laboratory and then returned to the patient either by the veins or as an injection under the skin. The therapy works by causing the immune system to recognize and attack the cancer cells.

ulcerative colitis: a type of inflammatory bowel disease. In this condition, the colon remains inflamed over a long period. This increases a person's risk for developing colon cancer, so starting colorectal cancer screening earlier and doing these tests more often is recommended.

ultrasound: an imaging method in which high-frequency sound waves are used to outline a part of the body. The sound wave echoes are picked up and displayed on a screen. In *intraoperative ultrasound,* the ultrasound is performed after a surgeon has opened the abdominal cavity. *Endorectal ultrasound* uses a special transducer that can be inserted directly into the rectum. Also called ultrasonography.

unproven therapy: any therapy that has not been scientifically tested and approved.

urostomy (you-RAHS-tuh-me): surgery to divert urine through a new passage and then through an opening in the abdomen. In a continent urostomy, the urine is stored inside the body and drained a few times a day through a tube placed into an opening called a stoma.

U.S. Food and Drug Administration (FDA): an agency of the United States Department of Health and Human Services. The FDA is responsible for regulating drugs, biological medical products, blood products, medical devices, and radiation-emitting devices, along with other products.

vascular endothelial (VAS-kyoo-lur en-doh-THEE-lee-uhl) growth factor (VEGF): a substance that stimulates the growth of new blood vessels.

virtual colonoscopy (ko-lun-AHS-kuh-pee): a noninvasive examination of the colon for polyps or cancer using special computerized tomography (CT) scans. The images are combined by a computer to create a 3-D model of the colon, which doctors can "fly through" on a computer screen. It is not yet clear if this new technique is as effective as other screening methods for colon cancer.

x-ray: one form of radiation that can be used at low levels to produce an image of the body on film or at high levels to destroy cancer cells.

Index

A

Abdomen, 4
Abdominoperineal resection, 92–93, 115, 116, 118
Ablation, types of
  ethanol (alcohol), 96
  laser, 119
  radiofrequency, 96, 112, 119
Abnormal growths, 5–8
Activity. *See* Physical activity
Acupuncture, 127, 128.
      See also Alternative
      and complementary
      therapies
Adenocarcinoma, 7
Adenomas, 6, 54, 55. *See also*
      Polyps
Adhesions, 94, 95
Adjuvant therapy, 77. *See*
      also Chemotherapy;
      Radiation therapy
African Americans, risk of
      colorectal cancer, 16
Age and colorectal cancer, 12,
      105, 107
AJCC (American Joint
      Committee on Cancer)
      staging system, 69–74
Alcohol, 17, 140
Allergic reaction to drugs,
      108–109
Alternative and comple-
      mentary therapies,
      127–131. *See also names*
      of specific therapies
American Cancer Society
  clinical trials matching
      service, 126–127
  document on anemia, 142
  document on chemo-
      therapy, 107
  document on clinical trials,
      127
  document on colostomies,
      89, 137
  document on fatigue, 142
  document on gastrointes-
      tinal carcinoid tumors, 7

document on gastrointes-
      tinal stromal tumors, 8
document on insurance, 58
document on non-Hodgkin
      lymphoma, 8
document on nutrition and
      physical activity, 28–29
document on sexuality and
      cancer, 95
early detection tests recom-
      mended by, 51–53
support resources from,
      145
telephone number, 7, 8, 29,
      58, 89, 95, 107, 127,
      130, 131, 137, 139,
      142, 145
tobacco cessation program,
      139
treatment guidelines, 131
Web site, 7, 8, 29, 58, 89,
      107, 123, 131, 137,
      142
American Joint Committee on
      Cancer (AJCC) staging
      system, 69–74
Amsterdam criteria, 25. *See*
      also Bethesda guidelines
Anastomosis, coloanal, 92
Anemia, 61, 142
Angiogenesis, 107
Angiogram, 68
Angiography, 68, 97
Antibody, monoclonal, 107.
      See also names of specific
      monoclonal antibodies
Anus, 4
APC gene, 14, 20, 21–22
Appendix, 4
Appetite, loss of, 106, 108
Ashkenazi Jews, risk of
      colorectal cancer, 16
Aspirin, 30–31, 150
Astler-Coller cancer staging
      system, 69, 74
Avastin (bevacizumab),
      107–108, 113, 118,
      152

B

Bethesda Criteria, 25–26
Bethesda guidelines, 25–26
Bevacizumab (Avastin),
    107–108, 113, 118,
    152
Bilirubin, elevated, 104
Biopsy, 34, 37, 62, 64
Bladder, and side effects of
    radiation therapy, 101
Bleeding. *See also* Blood in
    stool
  caused by NSAIDs, 30
  as side effect of chemo-
    therapy, 108
  as symptom, 60
  vulnerability to, 106
Blood cell counts, low, 104,
    106, 108
Blood in stool, 34, 38, 42–46,
    46–47, 60, 101
Blood tests, 60–61
Body weight, 27–29
Bowel, side effects on, 101
Bowel, small, 3–4
Bowel preparation
  for colonoscopy, 35–36, 37
  for computed tomography
    (CT) colonography, 41
  for double-contrast barium
    enema, 38–39
  for flexible sigmoidoscopy,
    33
  for surgery, 88, 91
Brachytherapy, 100, 114,
    115
Bruising, vulnerability to,
    106

C

Calcium, 29, 150
Camptosar (irinotecan),
    104–105, 108, 113,
    118, 152
Cancer, advanced, 102–103,
    104. *See also* Metastasis;
    Treatment by stage of
    disease; *names of specific
    sites of metastasis*
Cancer. *See also* Staging
    colorectal cancer
  definition of, 1, 3
  grade, 77, 83

  previous treatment for, as
    risk factor, 18–19
  spread of, 6–7
  start of, 6–7
Cancer care team, 79–86,
    133–134
Cancer cells, 1–2, 7, 83
Cancer Information Service
    (federal), 127
Cancer treatment as risk
    factor, 18–19
CA-19-9, 61, 137
Capecitabine (Xeloda),
    103–104, 105. *See also*
    CapeOX regimen
  for colon cancer, 110–111,
    113
  for rectal cancer, 116, 117,
    118
CapeOX regimen (capecit-
    abine and oxaliplatin),
    105
  for colon cancer, 111, 113
  for rectal cancer, 116, 117,
    118
Carcinoembryonic antigen,
    61, 137
Carcinogenesis, 21–22
Carcinoid tumors, 7
Carcinoma in situ, 70, 72
Causes of colorectal cancer,
    19–22
Causes of colorectal cancer as
    therapy targets, 107
CEA (carcinoembryonic
    antigen), 61, 137
Cecum, 4
Celecoxib (Celebrex) for
    polyp prevention, 30,
    150
Cells, cancer, 1–2, 7, 83
Cells, interstitial, of Cajal,
    7–8
Cetuximab (Erbitux),
    108–109, 113, 118, 152
Chemoprevention, 149–151
Chemotherapy, 101–107.
    See also Treatment by
    stage of disease; *names of
    specific drugs*
  adjuvant, 102, 105, 117
  for advanced cancer,
    102–103

drugs used in, 103–105
mechanism of, 105
neoadjuvant, 102, 116–117, 120
new drugs, 152
in recurrent rectal cancer, 119–120
regional, 101–102
side effects of, 103, 104, 105–107
systemic, 101
Chest x-ray, 67
Clinical stage, 68
Clinical trials, 121–127
American Cancer Society matching service, 126–127
definition of, 121
focus of, 121–122
information about, 126–127
informed consent in, 125
phases of, 122–124
questions to ask about, 126
in recurrent disease, 114, 120
risks of, 125
Web sites listing, 127
Colectomy, 88–90, 110–111
Colectomy, laparoscopic-assisted, 89–90
Colitis, ulcerative, 6, 12–13, 53
Coloanal anastamosis, 92
Colon, 4, 5, 71
Colonic J-pouch, 92
Colonoscope, 34–35, 36, 37, 38
Colonoscopy, 34–38, 49, 51, 52, 54, 55, 56, 57, 136, 137
Colonoscopy, virtual, 40–42, 50, 51, 64–65
Coloplasty, 92
Colostomy
averting, 116
to bypass tumor, 119
care for, 137
diverting, 112
permanent, 89, 93, 94

reversal, 89
temporary, 89, 92, 94
Communicating with health care providers, 133–134, 137–138
Complementary and alternative therapies, 127–131
Computed tomography, 40–42, 50, 51, 63–65
Consent, informed, 125
Constipation, 59
Control group, 124
Coping, 141
Counseling, genetic, 15–16, 21, 24–27
Crohn's disease, 6, 12–13, 53, 58
Cryosurgery, 97, 112, 119
CT (computed tomography), 40, 63–64
CT (computed tomography) colonography, 40–42, 50, 51, 64–65
Cyclooxygenase-2 inhibitors, 30–31, 150

D
Death, 2, 9, 17
Decisions about care, 87
Dendritic cells, 153
Detection of colorectal cancer or polyps. See also names of specific tests
American Cancer Society recommendations for early, 51–57
biopsy for, 62
early, 23–58, 151
imaging tests for, 62–68
for people at increased or high risk, 52–53, 54–57
Diabetes, type 2, 18
Diagnosis, 59–68
Diarrhea, 59, 101, 103, 104, 105, 108, 109
Diet and nutrition
and risk of colorectal cancer, 16–17, 27–29, 150–151
and recurrence, 143
and treatment, 139–140

Dietitian, 79
Digestive system, normal, 3–5
Digestive tract, 3, 5, 71
Digital rectal exam, 33, 36, 43, 51, 52, 60
DNA. *See also* Gene mutations
  damaged, and cancer, 1–2
  mutations, 19–22, 149
  in stool test, 47–48
Double-contrast barium enema, 38–40, 49, 51
DRE (digital rectal exam), 33, 36, 43, 51, 52, 60
Drugs. *See* Chemotherapy; *specific names of drugs and types of drugs*
Dukes cancer staging system, 69, 74
Dysplasia, 6, 54

E
Eating. *See* Diet and nutrition; Loss of appetite
Eloxatin (oxaliplatin), 105. *See also* CapeOX regimen; FOLFOX regimen
  in clinical trials, 152
  for colon cancer, 111, 113
  for rectal cancer, 116, 117, 118
Embolization, hepatic artery, 97–98
Emotional health, 141, 142, 143–145
Endocavitary radiation therapy, 99–100, 114, 115
Endometrial cancer, risk of, 15
Endorectal ultrasound, 66
Enterostomal therapist, 93, 137
Epidermal growth factor receptor, 108, 109
Erbitux (cetuximab), 108–109, 113, 118, 152
Ethanol (alcohol) ablation, 96
Examination, physical, 60, 68, 135, 136

Excision, local, 90
Exenteration, pelvic, 93, 116
Exercise, 17, 27–29, 140–142, 143
External beam radiation therapy, 99
Extracavitary radiation therapy, 99

F
Familial adenomatous polyposis. *See also* APC gene
  gene mutation and, 20, 24
  and risk of colorectal cancer, 14, 27, 53, 54, 57
  treating, 30, 150
Family. *See also* Resources
  health history and colorectal cancer, 13–14, 24–27, 53, 56, 57
  and screening schedule, 14, 53, 56, 57
  sharing good times with, 147
  as source of support, 144–145
Family history and screening, 14, 53, 56, 57
Fatigue, 60, 101, 106, 108, 109, 140–142
Fecal immunochemical test, 46–47, 50, 52, 151. *See also* Screening tests
Fecal occult blood test (FOBT), 42–46, 50, 51. *See also* Screening tests
Feces, definition of, 4
Fertility, effect of treatment on, 94–95
FIT (fecal immunochemical test), 46–47, 50, 52, 151. *See also* Screening tests
5-fluorouracil (5-FU), 103, 104, 111, 115, 118. *See also* FOLFIRI regimen; FOLFOX regimen
Five-year survival rate, 75, 76. *See also* Relative five-year survival rate

FOBT (fecal occult blood test), 42–46, 50, 51. *See also* Screening tests
FOLFIRI regimen (5-fluoro-uracil, leucovorin, and irinotecan), 104
  for colon cancer, 113
  for rectal cancer, 118
FOLFOX regimen (5-fluoro-uracil, leucovorin, and oxaliplatin), 105
  for colon cancer, 110–111, 113
  for rectal cancer, 115, 116, 117, 118
Folic acid, 17, 29, 150
Folinic acid. *See* Leucovorin
Fluorodeoxyglucose (FDG), 67
Fluorouracil (5-FU), 103, 104, 111, 115, 118. *See also* FOLFIRI regimen; FOLFOX regimen
Follow-up care, 135–137
Friends, support from, 144
Fruit-rich diet, 17, 27–28, 140
Full thickness resection, 91

G
Gadolinium, 66
Gardner syndrome, 14, 20
Gastroenterologist, 79–80
Gastrointestinal carcinoid tumors, 7
Gastrointestinal stromal tumors, 7–8
Gastrointestinal tract, 3–5, 71
Gene mutations, 19–22, 47, 149
Genetic counseling and testing, 15–16, 21, 24–27
Genetic counselor, 81
Grade of cancer, 77, 83
Growth of cells, abnormal, 1, 5–6, 21–22. *See also* Polyps
Guidelines
  screening, 51–57
  treatment, 131

H
Hair loss, 106
Headache, 108, 109
Health, lifestyle changes to improve, 138–142
Health care team, 79–86, 133–134
Hemicolectomy, 88–90, 110
Hepatic artery
  embolization, 97–98
  infusion, 102, 112, 118, 120
Hereditary nonpolyposis colon cancer (HNPCC), 14–15. *See also* Amsterdam criteria; Bethesda guidelines
  causes of, 20–21
  genetic testing and, 24–27
  screening and, 53, 54, 55, 57
  types of cancer associated with, 26–27
High-risk populations, 52–53, 54–57
History
  of colorectal cancer, 53, 55
  family health, 13–14, 53, 56, 57
  of polyps, 12, 53, 54–55
HNPCC. *See* Hereditary nonpolyposis colon cancer
Hope, maintaining, 147
Hormone replacement therapy, 31
Hospice, 146–147

I
I1307K APC mutation, 16. *See also* APC gene
Imaging tests, diagnostic, 62–68. *See also* Screening tests
  angiography, 68
  computed tomography, 63–64
  computed tomography (CT) colonography, 62, 64–65, 151

computed tomography (CT)–guided needle biopsy, 64
magnetic resonance imaging (MRI), 66–67
physician supervising, 84–85
positron emission tomography (PET), 67–68
ultrasound, 65–66
virtual colonoscopy, 62, 64–65, 151
x-ray, chest, 67
Imaging tests, follow-up, 135, 136
Immunotherapy, 152–153
Infection, vulnerability to, 106. *See also* Low blood cell counts
Inflammatory bowel disease, 12–13, 53, 57
Informed consent, 125
Inherited syndromes, 14–16
Insurance, 58, 138. *See also* Medicare
Intestinal tract, 3–5, 71
Intestine, large, 4
Intestine, small, 3–4
Intraoperative ultrasound, 66
Irinotecan (Camptosar), 104–105, 108, 113, 118, 152
Irritable bowel syndrome, 13

J
Jews, risk of colorectal cancer, 16

L
Laser therapy, 119
Leucovorin. *See also* FOLFIRI regimen; FOLFOX regimen
for colon cancer, 111, 113
with 5-FU, 103
with irinotecan, 104
with oxaliplatin, 105
for rectal cancer, 116, 117, 118
Lifestyle-related factors, 16–18, 138–142
Liver
chemotherapy for metastasis to, 102, 120
detecting disease in, 65, 66, 67
metastasis to, 112
treatment for metastasis to, 96–98, 111–113, 117–119
Local excision, 90, 91, 109–110, 114
Local transanal resection, 91, 115
Loneliness, coping with, 144–145
Loss of appetite, 106, 108
Low anterior resection, 91–92, 115, 116, 118
Low blood cell counts, 104, 106, 108
Lower GI series, 62
Lung, treatment for metastasis to, 111–113, 117–118
Lymphatic vessels, 6–7
Lymph nodes, 7, 8
Lymphoma, 8
Lynch syndrome. *See* Hereditary nonpolyposis colon cancer (HNPCC)

M
Magnesium, 29–30
Magnetic resonance imaging (MRI), in diagnosis, 66–67
Medical history, 60, 136
Medical oncologist, 81
Medical records, 137–138
Medicare, 58
Meditation, 128, 129
Melatonin, 18
Metastasis. *See also* Treatment by stage of disease; *names of specific sites of metastasis*
definition of, 2, 7
process of, 6–7
staging, 68–74
surgery for, 96–98
symptom-free, treatment for, 118
therapy for, 108, 111–113, 117–120
Metastases, surgical treatment of, 96–98

Monoclonal antibody, 107, 108, 109
Mortality, cancer, 2, 9
Mouth sores, 103, 106, 108
MRI (magnetic resonance imaging) in diagnosis, 66–67
Mucosa, 70, 71
Mucositis, 106, 108
Multivitamins, 29, 150
Muscularis mucosa, 70
Muscularis propria, 70

N

National Cancer Institute (NCI)
  Cancer Information Service, 127
  clinical trials listing, 127
  survival rate database, 75–76
  treatment guidelines, 131
National Comprehensive Cancer Network (NCCN) treatment guidelines, 131
Nausea. See also Vomiting
  and appetite loss, 139
  and chemotherapy, 103, 104, 106
  complementary therapies for, 128
  and radiation therapy, 100
Neoadjuvant therapy, 102
Night-shift work, 18
Nodes, staging disease in, 68–74
Nonsteroidal anti-inflammatory drugs (NSAIDs), 30–31, 150
Numbness, 105
Nurse practitioner, 82
Nurses, types of, 81–82
Nutrition, 16–17, 27–29, 139–140, 150–151

O

Obesity, 17, 28
Oncogene, 19
Oncologist, medical, 81
Oncology-certified nurse, 82
Ovaries, treatment for metastasis to, 111–113

Oxaliplatin (Eloxatin), 105. See also CapeOX regimen; FOLFOX regimen
  in clinical trials, 152
  for colon cancer, 111, 113
  for rectal cancer, 116, 117, 118

P

Pain, 60, 82–83, 99, 146
Pain specialist, 82–83
Palliative care, 112, 118–119, 146–147
Panitumumab (Vectibix), 109, 113, 118, 152
Pathologic stage, 68–69
Pathologist, 62, 83
Patient-physician communication, 133–134, 137–138
PEI (percutaneous ethanol injection), 96
Pelvic exenteration, 93, 116
Percutaneous ethanol injection (PEI), 96
Peritoneum, treatment for metastasis to, 111–113
PET (positron emission tomography), 67–68
PET (positron emission tomography)/CT (computed tomography) scan, 67–68
Peutz-Jeghers syndrome, 15, 21
Phases of clinical trials, 122–124
Photocoagulation, 119
Physical activity, 17, 27–29, 140–142, 143
Physical examination, 60, 68, 135, 136
Physician, primary care, 83
Physician assistant, 83
Physician-patient communication, 133–134, 137–138
Polypectomy, 34, 37, 90, 91, 109–110, 114
Polyps, 6. See also Screening tests
  preventing, 30, 150

removal of, 34, 37, 90, 91,
    109–110, 114
  as risk factor, 12, 13–16,
    53, 54–55
  as start of cancer, 6
  tests to detect, 31–68
  types of, 6
Portal vein, 64
Positron emission tomog-
    raphy (PET), 67–68
Post-treatment care, 135–138
Prevention, colorectal cancer,
    23–31, 149–151.
    See also Screening
    for colorectal cancer;
    Screening tests
Prognosis, factors affecting,
    18
Psychiatrist, 84. *See also*
    Emotional health;
    Patient-physician
    communication
Psychologist, 84. *See also*
    Emotional health;
    Patient-physician
    communication

Q
Quality of life, 146
Questions for health care
    team, 133–134. *See
    also* Patient-physician
    communication

R
Radiation oncologist, 84
Radiofrequency ablation, 96,
    112, 119
Radiologist, 84–85
Rash, 109
Radiation therapy, 98–101.
    See also Side effects;
    *names of specific types of
    radiation therapy*
  adjuvant, 111, 114, 117,
    120
  brachytherapy, 100, 115
  endocavitary, 99–100
  external beam, 99
  internal, 100
  as neoadjuvant therapy,
    116–117
  physician supervising, 84

as risk factor, 18–19
  side effects of, 100–101
  for symptom control, 99
Radiofrequency ablation, 96,
    112, 119
Rectum
  bleeding from, 60
  hyperplastic polyps of, 54
  side effects that affect the,
    101
  surgery for cancer of, 90–93
  treatment for cancer of, by
    stage, 114–120
Recurrence, cancer
  and diet, 143
  distant, 113–114, 120
  fear of, 135
  follow-up care and,
    135–137
  local, 113, 119–120
  and physical activity, 143
  reducing risk of, 142–143
  tests for, 136–137
  therapy for, 113–114,
    119–120
Registered nurse, 81–82
Research, recent colorectal
    cancer, 149–153
  chemoprevention, 149–151
  on earlier detection, 151
  genetics, 149
  on new treatments,
    152–153
Resection. *See also* Surgery;
    *specific names of surgical
    procedures*
  abdominoperineal, 92–93,
    115, 116, 118
  colon, 110
  full thickness, 91
  low anterior, 91–92, 115,
    116, 118
  segmental, 88–89, 112
  transanal, 91, 114, 115,
    116
Rest, 140–142
Risk, increased or high,
    screening recommenda-
    tions for, 54–57
Risk factors, colorectal cancer,
    11–19
  age, 12
  family health history, 13–14

history of polyps, 12
inflammatory bowel disease, 12-13
inherited syndromes, 14–16
lifestyle-related factors, 16–18
racial and ethnic background, 16
uncertain, 18–19
Risk of cancer or cancer recurrence, 3, 8, 142–143, 149–151

S
Screening for colorectal cancer, 23–24. *See also* Counseling, genetic; Testing, genetic; Screening tests
guidelines for, 51–57
insurance coverage of, 58
for those with family history of adenomatous polyps, 56
for those with family history of colorectal cancer, 56
for those with increased risk, 19, 54-57
for those with inherited syndromes, 15–16
Screening tests, 31–50
colonoscopy, 34–38, 49, 51, 52, 54, 55, 56, 57, 136, 137
CT colonography, 40–42, 50, 51, 64–65
double-contrast barium enema, 38–40, 49, 51
fecal immunochemical test, 46–47, 50, 52, 151
fecal occult blood test, 42–46, 50, 51
pros and cons of various, 49–50
recommendations for people at average risk, 51–52
recommendations for people at high risk, 54–57
side effects of, 34, 37–38, 40, 42

sigmoidoscopy, flexible, 32–34, 49, 51
stool DNA tests, 47–48, 50, 52
sDNA (stool DNA) tests, 47–48, 50, 52
Segmental resection, 88–89, 112
Serosa, 70, 71
Sexual function, impact of treatment on, 94–95, 101
Side effects. *See also names of specific side effects*
of bevacizumab (Avastin), 108
of capecitabine (Xeloda), 104
of cetuximab (Erbitux), 108–109
of chemotherapy, 105–107
duration of, 101, 106
of 5-fluorouracil (5-FU), 103
of irinotecan (Camptosar), 104–105
of oxaliplatin (Eloxatin), 105
of panitumumab (Vectibix), 109
of radiation therapy, 100–101
reducing, ways of, 106–107
of surgery, 93–95
Sigmoidoscope, 32, 33, 34
Sigmoidoscopy, flexible, 32–34, 49, 51
Signs and symptoms of colorectal cancer, 59–60
Skin
and side effects of chemotherapy, 103, 104
and side effects of radiation therapy, 100
Smoking, 17, 61
cessation, 139
Social support, 143–144
Social worker, 85
Spread of cancer, 6–7
Stage, cancer, 5, 68–74
Stage grouping, 72–74
Staging colorectal cancer, 68–74

American Joint Committee on Cancer system, 69–74
Astler-Coller system, 69, 74
clinical, 68
comparison of systems, 74
Dukes system, 69, 74
I–IV, samples of, 72–74
pathologic, 68–69
stage grouping, 72–74
TNM (tumor, node, metastasis) system, 69–72
Stages I–IV, samples of, 72–74. See also Treatment by stage of disease
Statistics, colorectal cancer, 8–9
Stent, 112, 119
Stoma, 89
Stool, definition of, 4
Stool DNA test, 47–48, 50, 52
Stool, tests for colorectal cancer in, 42–48, 50, 51, 52
Submucosa, 70, 71
Subserosa, 70, 71
Survival rates for colorectal cancer, 75–77
Sunlight, sensitivity to, 103, 109
Support, emotional, 143–144
Surgeon, 85–86
Surgery, 87–98. See also Resection; specific names of surgical procedures
colon, 88–90
for metastasis, 96–98
physician performing, 85–86
rectal, 90–93
sexual function, impact on, 94–95
side effects of, 93–95
Survival rates, 75–77
extending, with chemotherapy, 102–103
Symptoms and signs of colorectal cancer, 59–60
Syndromes, inherited, 14–16

T

Talking with health care team, 133–134, 137–138

Targeted therapy, 107–109, 152
Testing, genetic, 15–16, 21, 24–27
Therapy, adjuvant, 77. See also Chemotherapy; Radiation therapy
Therapy, neoadjuvant, 102, 112, 116, 117, 119
Therapy, targeted, 107–109, 152
Therapy, tests of new. See Clinical trials
Tingling, in extremities, 105
TNM (tumor, node, metastasis) staging system, 69–72
Tobacco use, 17, 61, 139
Transanal resection, 91, 114, 115, 116
Treatment, 79–131. See also Chemotherapy; Clinical trials; Complementary and alternative therapies; Immunotherapy; Radiation therapy; Resection; Surgery; Therapy, targeted; Treatment by stage of disease; specific names of therapies
failure of, 145–147
guidelines, 131
methods of, 87
new, 152–153
targeted, 107–109
Treatment by stage of disease
for colon cancer, 109–114
for rectal cancer, 114–120
recurrent, 113–114 (colon), 119–120 (rectal)
stage 0, 109–110 (colon), 114 (rectal)
stage I, 110 (colon), 115 (rectal)
stage II, 110–111 (colon), 115–116 (rectal)
stage III, 111 (colon), 116–117 (rectal)
stage IV, 111–113 (colon), 117–119 (rectal)
Treatment guidelines, 131

Treatment types. *See* Chemo-
    therapy; Complementary
    and alternative therapies;
    Immunotherapy;
    Radiation therapy;
    Resection; Surgery;
    Therapy, targeted; *specific
    names of therapies*
Tumor
    benign, 2, 5–6
    cancer formation as, 2
    carcinoid, 7
    gastrointestinal stromal, 7–8
Tumor markers, 61, 137
Tumor suppressor genes, 19

U
Ulcerative colitis, 6, 12–13,
    53, 57
Ultrasound, 65–66
Urologist, 86
Urostomy, 93

V
Vaccines, tumor, 152–153
Vascular endothelial growth
    factor (VEGF), 107
Vectibix (panitumumab),
    109, 113, 118, 152

Vegetable-rich diet, 17,
    27–28, 140
Virtual colonoscopy, 40–42,
    50, 51, 64–65
Vitamins, 29, 150
Vomiting, 106. *See also*
    Nausea

W
Walking, 141, 143
Web resources
    for clinical trials, 127
    for treatment guidelines,
    131
Weight, body, 27–29. *See also*
    Obesity
Weight loss, 139–140. *See
    also* Appetite, loss of

X
Xeloda (capecitabine),
    103–104, 105. *See also*
    CapeOX regimen
    for colon cancer, 110–111,
    113
    for rectal cancer, 116, 117,
    118
x-ray, 38, 39, 67

Books Published
by the American Cancer Society

Available everywhere books are sold and online at
www.cancer.org/bookstore

Cancer Information

General

The Cancer Atlas (available in English, Spanish, French, Chinese)

Cancer: What Causes It, What Doesn't

The Tobacco Atlas, Second Edition (available in English, Spanish, French)

Information for People with Cancer

Site-Specific

ACS's Complete Guide to Colorectal Cancer

ACS's Complete Guide to Prostate Cancer

Breast Cancer Clear & Simple: All Your Questions Answered

QuickFACTS™ Advanced Cancer

QuickFACTS™ Bone Metastasis

QuickFACTS™ Lung Cancer

QuickFACTS™ Prostate Cancer

Praise for *QuickFACTS™ Lung Cancer*:
"The ACS has achieved its goal of providing overviews
that tackle need-to-know issues and supply references for
additional follow-up information as desired.
Recommended."
—Library Journal

Symptoms and Side Effects

ACS's Guide to Pain Control, Revised Edition

Eating Well, Staying Well During and After Cancer

Lymphedema: Understanding and Managing Lymphedema After Cancer Treatment

Support for Families and Caregivers

Cancer Caregiving A to Z: An At-Home Guide for Patients and Families

Cancer in the Family: Helping Children Cope with a Parent's Illness

Caregiving: A Step-by-Step Resource for Caring for the Person with Cancer at Home, Revised Edition

Couples Confronting Cancer: Keeping Your Relationship Strong

Get Better! Communication Cards for Kids & Adults (bilingual communication cards)

Social Work in Oncology: Supporting Survivors, Families, and Caregivers

When the Focus Is on Care: Palliative Care and Cancer

Help for Children

Because . . . Someone I Love Has Cancer: Kids' Activity Book (5 twist-up crayons included)

Mom and the Polka-Dot Boo-Boo

Our Dad Is Getting Better

Our Mom Has Cancer (available in hard cover and paperback)

Our Mom Is Getting Better

Health Books for Children

Healthy Air: A Read-Along Coloring & Activity Book (25 per pack; Tobacco avoidance)

Healthy Bodies: A Read-Along Coloring & Activity Book (25 per pack; Physical activity)

Healthy Food: A Read-Along Coloring & Activity Book (25 per pack; Nutrition)

Healthy Me: A Read-Along Coloring & Activity Book

Kids' First Cookbook: Delicious-Nutritious Treats to Make Yourself!

Tools for the Health Conscious

ACS's Healthy Eating Cookbook, Third Edition

Celebrate! Healthy Entertaining for Any Occasion

Good for You! Reducing Your Risk of Developing Cancer

The Great American Eat-Right Cookbook

Kicking Butts: Quit Smoking and Take Charge of Your Health

National Health Education Standards: Achieving Excellence, Second Edition (available in paperback and on CD-ROM)

Inspirational Survivor Stories

Angels & Monsters: A child's eye view of cancer

Crossing Divides: A Couple's Story of Cancer, Hope, and Hiking Montana's Continental Divide

I Can Survive (Illustrated)*

*A "Mom's Choice Awards" Finalist! (2007)